ON THE
EDGE OF LIFE:
Diary of A Medical
Intensive Care Unit

MIKKAEL A. SEKERES, M.D., M.S.,
and
THEODORE A. STERN, M.D.

Addresses for Correspondence:

Mikkael A. Sekeres, M.D., M.S.
Director, Leukemia Program
Professor of Medicine
Cleveland Clinic Taussig Cancer Institute
Cleveland, Ohio USA
Tel: 216-445-9353
Fax: 216-636-0636
Email: sekerem@ccf.org

Theodore A. Stern, M.D.
Chief, Avery D. Weisman Psychiatry Consultation Service,
Massachusetts General Hospital
Director, Office for Clinical Careers, Massachusetts General Hospital
Ned H. Cassem Professor of Psychiatry in the field of Psychosomatic
Medicine/Consultation,
Harvard Medical School
Boston, Massachusetts USA
Tel: 617-724-1520
Fax: 617-726-5946
Email: TStern@Partners.org

DEDICATION

To all of the people who have inspired me throughout my life: My teachers and students; all of my patients; and of course, my parents and the rest of my family, Jennifer, Gabriel, Samantha, and Silas.

— Mikkael A. Sekeres, M.D., M.S.

To my mentors, my colleagues, my students, and my patients and their families … who have faced critical illness and who have performed at their best and at their worst … with the hope that compassionate and excellent care will flow from enhanced awareness and understanding.

— Theodore A. Stern, M.D.

TABLE OF CONTENTS

About this Book

The entries recorded in the seven-volume "Medical Intensive Care Unit (MICU) Journal" cover a twenty-year period, beginning in January, 1980. They reflect the musings of Interns, Junior Assistant Residents (or, "JARs"), and Senior Assistant Residents (or, "SARs") in the Internal Medicine Residency Training Program at the Massachusetts General Hospital (MGH). We have taken the liberty of reorganizing the entries into chapters based on common themes (e.g., "Humor", "Life and Death"), thereby violating their chronology. Within chapters, too, we have tried to organize entries based on common threads (e.g., within the "Humor" chapter, jokes related to urinary catheters have been placed together). Our intent was to enable the reader to complete entire chapters in a single sitting.

As a further aid to readers who do not work in health care, we have created a running glossary that defines medical terms and jargon unique to the field of medicine. Any term bolded in an entry is defined and placed for quick reference in an alphabetical glossary at the back of the book.

We have also weighed-in with our own comments after one or more entries or following a particularly jarring statement. These comments appear as italicized text. In doing so, we have attempted to provide a common voice that can be heard throughout the book, placing some entries in a larger context and making sense of some of the more obtuse entries. Our intent was to make these interjections as unobtrusive as possible.

Finally, to preserve the anonymity of both the patients and the physicians who have passed through the MICU, each date has been modified: sometimes by a few months, sometimes by several years. In addition, the diseases afflicting certain patients and on occasion even the gender of a patient or doctor has been changed to maintain the confidentiality and recognizability of a person or situation. In all other ways, the content of the entries is unaltered from how it appeared in the actual journal.

The doctors who wrote in the journal had no idea their entries, which reflect the MICU-related experiences of the young physicians, would be published eventually. As a result their stories, humor, and reflections are honest and recorded in real time. It should be noted that every physician whose entry was included in this volume has provided consent for inclusion in this book. Sometimes raw, sometimes somber, we hope these musings provide insights into the often surreal life of the MICU.

Mikkael A. Sekeres, M.D., M.S.
Theodore A. Stern, M.D.

Foreword

In 1978, I began working in the Medical Intensive Care Unit (MICU) at the Massachusetts General Hospital (MGH). As the psychiatric consultant to the MICU, I attended medical rounds and provided direct patient care. In addition to these functions, I also worked with the residents themselves. Having seen the benefits of a weekly seminar on self-awareness for psychiatry residents (conducted at the MGH by Dr. Edward Messner), I created similar rounds, called autognosis rounds, for the medical house staff in the MICU. Autognosis (meaning self-awareness) refers to a clinician's knowledge and to the ways in which that knowledge affects his or her interactions with patients and colleagues.

Discussion of clinical problems, residents' reactions to such problems, and review of the literature relating to countertransference (an emotional reaction to the patient determined by the physician's own unconscious conflicts) formed the core of Messner's seminar. However, a somewhat different approach was required when working with medical house staff (physicians-in-training). By the very nature of their training, medical interns and residents spend less of their workweek focused on self-observation than do psychiatrists-in-training. Yet, they as a group are still vulnerable to disappointment, anxiety, fear, insecurity, grief, and anger. Their work with critically ill individuals places them squarely in the midst of pain, delirium, and death. These factors, as well as endless demands, long work hours, and profound sleep deprivation set the stage for experiencing intense emotions.

Since 1978, more than 500 house officers have rotated through the MICU and attended autognosis rounds; only a handful has refused to participate. Rounds have several goals. First, to help residents identify their reactions to clinical situations. Second, to help residents learn how to use their emotions in clinical settings (e.g., by recognizing that a resident's apprehension experienced during the admission work-up of a 55-year-old man, who looks and sounds like her father, might be stimulated by her reaction to the patient, who reminds her of her father). Third, to learn how to minimize potentially disruptive effects of their reactions (e.g., anger) to patients. Fourth, to have residents share their reactions with each other and to learn that they are not alone with their feelings. Humor and the use of metaphor help residents learn about the autognostic process.

Typically, I would introduce rounds as follows: "Auto means self or car. Gnosis means knowledge or awareness. So auto-gnosis involves knowing yourself or knowing your car. Just imagine what would happen if you only looked straight ahead while you were driving (that would be like paying attention only to a patient's laboratory data). You'd get sideswiped. But, if you only focused on the images in your rear-view and side-view mirrors (which would be like paying exclusive attention to your feelings and to those of your patients) you'd get into a head-on collision. Safe driving requires looking at both the road and the mirrors (data and feelings). The more you know about your car (or self) the better prepared you will be. Driving conditions change and you need to know a good mechanic to whom you can turn when accidents (or problems) occur. You need to know how to change gears, directions, and speed, and how to signal; remember to keep a close eye on your fuel (or sustenance/support) gauge." Based on my use of this metaphor, rounds were often called "Car Rounds."

Rounds generally involved discussion of cases (e.g., irritation with a 42-year-old non-MGH physician who began [inappropriately] writing orders in his father's MICU medical record), the use of fantasy, and the use of likeability scales. Most important was the encouragement of self-awareness, which a physician must have to practice medicine well. For example, on one occasion I was called to the emergency room to see an agitated young man wearing an Army fatigue jacket, because he was making threatening (martial arts) gestures to passerbys; this behavior prompted the Boston Police to bring him to the hospital. When I met him he was seated on a stretcher with his legs draped over the side rail. After several minutes I noticed that I adopted a protective stance with my hands in front of my genitals, and I realized that his pointed cowboy boots were in striking distance of my groin. My thoughts shifted to a hiking trip I had taken in the Grand Tetons with my wife, where we had been chased and treed by a bear. This memory of feeling vulnerable and terrified, and the link I made between the two situations, prompted me to excuse myself from the patient's room. I returned with members of the hospital's security force, who ensured my safety during the evaluation. While I should have known from the outset that I was in danger, it took my recollection of the encounter with the bear to realize it. Awareness of my apprehension enabled me to protect myself and to provide an appropriate assessment of the patient.

It was apparent during the first year of these rounds that some residents were more comfortable than others when talking about their reactions to patients. I thought that for those who were reluctant it might be easier for them to express their feelings in writing. Therefore, in 1980, as a supplement to autognosis rounds, I created the "Red Book," so named because of the book's red cover. Members of the MICU team were encouraged to record their thoughts and feelings that were stimulated by their MICU work. The initial entry included the statement, "Anonymous or not, the thrills and spills you provide (both cognitive and affective) are welcome."

Providing humane care in the ICU is a challenge; the work is highly technological and is often complicated by noises, distractions, and interruptions. Someone is always doing something to someone in the ICU, and physicians must care for patients despite physical and pharmacological barriers. Tubes placed down a patient's windpipe enable a mechanical ventilator to do the work of breathing but prevent him from speaking. Paralytic drugs allow a patient to be ventilated without resistance, while sedatives alleviate anxiety and fear yet also may cause confusion. Without question, the ICU experience is emotionally intense and physically draining. Work in the ICU is reminiscent of scenes portrayed on "House," "Scrubs," "ER" or "M*A*S*H*," but life in the MICU does not follow a script.

Medical records in the MICU are voluminous; data pour in hour by hour. Notes from ICU staff, consultants, respiratory therapists, nurses, and caregivers from outside hospitals are continuously added to the chart. Highly complex ICU flow sheets - originally on paper, now electronic - are kept that include graphic representations of physiologic parameters (e.g., blood pressure, heart rate, respiratory rate, temperature, pupillary size, fluid balance [including the amount and types of all fluids going in and out of the patient], laboratory values, medications ordered and administered, and observations about the patient's behavior). Reviewing these flow sheets requires keen eyesight; each day's worksheet is equivalent to six sheets of paper folded together. Column after column is filled in with the products of hour-by-hour data entry. A single change in any data point can have dramatic consequences. For example, an increase in the creatinine (a measure of kidney function) might mean that all medications excreted by the kidneys may need to be adjusted. If the results of an arterial blood gas (ABG) show a decrease in the oxygenation of the blood, oxygen may need to be administered, fluid overload may need to be addressed, or the patient may need to be placed on a ventilator. In addition, results of repeated physical examinations and assessments are documented several times each day.

The fast-paced action of the ICU often bonds staff. This is part of the appeal for those who work in the ICU.... a battlefield camaraderie. Unfortunately, these same factors also place them at risk for "burnout" and distress. Though many MICU patients are near death, they do not lie quietly. Rather, they often become agitated or threatening, risking injury to themselves or to the staff; appropriate measures must be taken to ensure everyone's safety. Mechanical restraints used in combination with some degree of sedation are typically employed when the threat is serious. MICU patients suffer from anxiety, fear, agitation, depression, dread, despondency, helplessness, and thoughts of suicide; each can lead to increased morbidity, disability, and mortality.

Some patients become convinced that they are going to die even when their doctors don't think that they will. At these times, education may ward off catastrophic reactions. Empathy and support are helpful. Patients have concerns about the comfort and autonomy, and the availability of their loved ones; they also fear that they'll be abandoned by their caregivers.

Personality styles are often magnified in the ICU. Many patients fall back on familiar (maladaptive) behavior patterns when stressed by severe illness; it is their best or only line of defense. For example, the paranoid person becomes more hostile, suspicious, and convinced that others are trying to poison them.

Treatment with mechanical ventilation is typically associated with anxiety. Moreover, the experience of having a tube down one's throat is uncomfortable and frightening. Even after extubation (removal of the tube), the patient finds that his respiratory muscles have become deconditioned from disuse. Thus, one can feel unable to catch one's breath, and this creates more anxiety. Moreover, the constant rhythmic noise of the mechanical ventilator and the feeling that one is repeatedly trying to breathe against resistance (like blowing up a balloon that is two-thirds full) drives some people to distraction.

When alert, patients worry about what will happen to them, and often will be unable to be reassured. Staff members, burdened by concerns about critical illness and their reluctance to be the bearers of bad news to patients and families, will sometimes withdraw or direct their frustration, anger, and helplessness towards colleagues, patients, and families. They are stressed by sleep deprivation, long duty hours, limited training in ethical dilemmas, exposure to infectious diseases, complex presentations of medical and neuropsychiatric illness, information overload, and by concerns about malpractice. In addition, they have concerns about dying, inflicting pain, prolonging life, and by environmental disruptions, administrative conflicts, and unpredictable schedules.

Measures used to reduce a patient's suffering or fear are often overlooked or are inadequate. Nurses regularly provide reassurance and reorientation; visits by frustrated and frightened families and friends, may be helpful, but more often than not this exhausts already sleep-deprived patients. Environmental manipulations (e.g., turning on and off lights to approximate the day and night cycles) rarely reverse the confusion so often encountered in the ICU.

Although history-taking is relatively straightforward throughout most of the hospital, this is not the case with an agitated or intubated ICU patient. Most physicians lack the ability to read lips or to interpret hand gestures (which are often hampered by the use of restraints, intravenous [IV] lines, or arterial catheters in the wrists). In the ICU, communication is often too slow and inadequate for the pace and problems at hand. To address these limitations in communication, physicians and nurses may limit their inquires to "yes" and "no" questions aimed at symptom identification. Use of a letter board (where one can point to one letter at a time to spell out words) is helpful, but painstakingly slow.

One may ask, more than 30 years after the book was created, (though its cover is no longer red) whether the MICU diary is still relevant, or necessary. We would argue, without doubt, a resounding "Yes!" MICU's have become even more technological, complicated places than ever before, and the patients have become sicker, as previous MICU inhabitants have become increasingly treated on regular medical floors. Residents, staff physicians, mid-levels, and nurses have become no less vulnerable. It continues to attract insightful, often prolific, entries. As you read the diary entries included here, try to remember that work in the MICU occurs at an uneven pace. The tone and lengths of entries in the MICU diary (written by hundreds of house officers) reflect this. Philosophy, outrage, horror, and humor coexist. While hundreds have made entries, a single voice is often heard from their common experience. The conflicts that arose for house officers in the 1980s and 90s continue to be problematic for residents today. Although the technology of the MICU has advanced, residents still struggle with matters of life and death, with family dynamics, and with poor prognoses associated with critical illness.

The MICU is not always civilized; our hope is that readers will come to appreciate how the stresses and strains of MICU work both nurture and corrupt young physicians. A word of caution: be prepared to ride the roller coaster with the staff in the MICU. Try to withhold premature judgment, as their experiences seep into your consciousness. As you will soon see, life in the MICU is certainly not normal.

Theodore A. Stern, M.D.

Introduction

At 7:00 AM on June 26, 1996, my first day of internship at the Massachusetts General Hospital (MGH), I entered the Medical Intensive Care Unit (MICU) to begin my first rotation. And I was scared out of my wits. Somehow, during four years of medical school in Philadelphia, I had managed to avoid any intensive care unit (ICU) rotations, and had no idea what to expect. I pushed the big silver button on the wall outside the MICU to open the automatic doors, walked through, and was struck at first by the sounds: medication machines beeping in sets of three ("Bing-bing, bong; bing-bing, bong") to notify the nurses that a medication had run out or that an IV line was kinked; cardiac monitors for each patient recording normal heart rhythms ("Bee-boop, bee-boop, bee-boop…bomp") or warning of abnormal ones ("Ring! Ring! Ring!"); the ventilators alarming (during periods when patients stopped breathing) in one, long, continuous screech ("Meeeeeeeeeeeeeeehhhh!"); and the janitor buffing the floors ("Rumm-ah-rumm-ah-rumm-ah-rumm"). Within a few days, I could close my eyes and identify every sound and know which were serious and which I could ignore. I adapted, and treated the sounds like white noise (though when I spoke to my parents from the phone at the nurse's station, they always reminded me how much the cacophony still bothered them).

That first day, when I was still an outsider, I just wanted to stare at the patients who occupied the 17 beds in the MICU. However, I thought it would be impolite. And I found myself staring anyway. As I walked past room after room, faces and bodies flashed by in succession like the slow-motion images of a battle scene from a war movie. Mostly old bodies, the majority with their mouths cocked-open around clear plastic breathing tubes, they each had IV lines entering their necks and chests, as well as their arms. As many as 10 medication pumps hung on a bar behind the beds of some patients. Each patient had a urine bag, some had rectal bags, and some had wrist restraints in place to prevent the accidental removal of the breathing tube in a fit of consciousness. And each one was sedated. Otherwise, how else could they tolerate this technology? Some of their rooms, though, had a touch of humanity: the crayon or watercolor drawings on the bulletin board wishing "Get well soon, Granpa!" or the photographs at family reunions. Or the rosaries.

As interns (the first year of a three-year residency in internal medicine), we "rotated" onto different services in the hospital, spending one month in the MICU, then one month on an inpatient service, then one month on an outpatient practice, and so on. I was informed that I would be on-call my first night. What does it mean to be a resident "on-call"? First I should describe the resident team structure, and how a typical day in the MICU goes. Four interns rotate through the MICU each month. Each intern is paired with a second-year resident (also called a Junior Admitting Resident, or "JAR"), and that duo is responsible for the care of a given number of patients (typically 4-6). Two sets of intern-junior pairs report to a third-year resident (a Senior Admitting Resident, or "SAR"), and the two seniors report to an attending (the boss – a physician who has completed all of his or her training), and a Pulmonary & Critical Care fellow (a fellowship begins after one has completed the three years of residency, for those who want to specialize further within medicine). All together, this group makes up the team of doctors who staff the MICU each month and, with the nurses and other providers such as respiratory therapists, care for 14-17 extremely sick patients.

The group of four interns, four juniors, and two seniors, along with any medical students rotating through the MICU, gathers in a windowless conference room at 7:00 a.m. to review the events of the previous night. They look at the patients' vital signs and other data (heart rate, blood pressure, respiratory rate, temperature, ventilator settings, and medication drip rates); procedures performed; test results; and notable occurrences (e.g., one patient started vomiting blood; another no longer requires the high-dose cardiac medications to keep her blood pressure up; a third died). These "sign-in rounds" take about 45 minutes, after which each intern-junior pair rounds on their patients. They examine them, record their vital signs, write a daily progress note, and with the nurse also caring for that patient, formulate the plan for the day.

At 10:00 a.m. the entire team (now including the attending, the fellow, and the nurses) gathers around a cart (which contains the patients' medical records) or around a gaggle of "computers on wheels" or "COWs" and push them from room-to-room while discussing each patient. These rounds can last 2-3 hours, but have even extended until as late as 4:30 or 5:00 in the afternoon. Around noon the entire group gathers in the tiny conference room for a lecture and lunch, after which the team disperses and the intern-junior pairs do the work of caring for their patients: ordering tests, drawing blood, calling specialists (e.g., the patient vomiting blood requires a gastroenterologist; the cardiologist needs an update on the patient who no longer requires high-dose cardiac medications). At the end of the day ("end" being defined loosely), the group gathers again in the conference room for "sign-out rounds," during which three intern-junior pairs tell the fourth, the on-call pair, how to manage their patients overnight.

Obviously, a resident cannot remain in the hospital every hour of every day to care for his or her patients. Yet these patients are so sick, they require constant observation. Nurses work traditional eight or twelve-hour shifts and are responsible for only 1-2 patients at a time. They "give report" on patient events to the next nurse coming on shift. Residents spend one in every four nights in the hospital on-call, following an ordinary work day, caring for everybody's patients and admitting new patients, whose care they assume subsequent to that night. A resident will average 1-2 hours of sleep on those nights; often he or she will not get any. The on-call team then reports that night's events to the rest of the team during sign-in rounds. All told, when on-call, a resident spends about 32 hours straight in the hospital.

When rotating through the MICU, interns and residents get about 2 days off a month, usually working 90-100 hours per week.

To prepare for my first day and night, I packed my stethoscope, reflex hammer, ophthalmoscope, reference books, a brand new white coat, and a slew of pens, as well as my glasses and contact lens case, a comb, and a change of underwear. Sadly, the last two would go unused. At sign-in rounds, the post-call intern-junior pair from the previous group gave report on all the patients. My junior, Dave, brought them breakfast – it is a tradition, I learned, that the on-call team always brings the post-call team food in the morning. We dispersed to round on our patients: an 85-year-old woman who had been in the hospital for two months with pneumonia complicated by destruction of her lungs; a 74-year-old man with a devastating stroke leaving him paralyzed on the right and unable to speak or to understand questions; and a 45-year-old man with low blood pressure awaiting a liver transplant. I started to ask the first woman how she was feeling before realizing she couldn't answer with the ventilator tube in her mouth. So much for substantive patient interactions. We examined the patients together, fighting the cardiac monitor leads and IV lines with our stethoscopes. I struggled to figure out how to read the flow sheets of vital signs while Dave wrote the progress note for the day and dictated the plan. He also showed me how to use the computer system. I felt like an infant – everything I experienced was new, and I could do little to help Dave with the day's work.

Rounds with the attending and fellow lasted three hours – I spent a lot of the time leaning against a wall, and my sleeves were filthy by the end of the day! The attending took a few digressions to teach pulmonary mechanics and ventilator management strategies, some of which I remembered from med school, but most of which, again, were new. The junior and senior residents digressed a few times to crack jokes, trying to relieve the tension. The interns were far too terrified, though, to do much more than smile uncomfortably! After hearing that a patient was on four antibiotics, one senior commented, "Well,

I guess we have everything covered, except maybe maggots!" When the attending asked how a severely demented man with a widespread infection was doing, the junior caring for him quipped, "Much better, though I still wouldn't want him as my Quiz Bowl partner…"

Following rounds, we had pizza for lunch. That afternoon, Dave showed me how to place an arterial line into a patient and I wrote my first order as a physician (to give a patient potassium). Actually, the nurse told me the patient needed potassium, taught me how to write the order, what to give, where, and when. But I was able to sign my name without any help! Probably half my education as an intern (and much more than half that first month) I received from the nurses, who knew how to care for patients a lot better than I. Before long, at about 7:00 p.m., we reconvened for sign-out rounds, during which we sat with the list of patients and assiduously listed all of the tasks the other intern-junior teams gave us to perform on their patients that night. Everyone else left for the evening, and we were alone.

Alone. I know that during times of extreme terror people can remember every detail of an experience and it never leaves them, but a lot of that night is now a blur. Astutely (as I did not have a clue what I was doing), Dave sent me on errands while he stayed in the Unit to manage the patients. I went down to the cafeteria at 9:00 p.m. to grab dinner for us (another tradition at MGH is that all residents gather at 9:00 p.m., when the cafeteria is closed to the public, for a communal meal), saw some of my co-interns to whom I gave a resigned wave, and headed back up to the Unit. I was sent on a journey to the largely abandoned radiology department to find some X-rays and quickly got lost along unlit hallways. I also escorted a newly-ventilated patient from the Emergency Room back up to the Unit and wondered what I would do if, God forbid, he coded (i.e., had a cardiac arrest) in the elevator.

I remember running into a couple of patients' rooms with Dave when those patients suddenly dropped their blood pressures that night, and into another room when a man became short of breath.

"What's the matter?" Dave asked.

"Can't…breathe." We got a stat X-ray of his chest (the radiologists roll a large machine into a patient's room and snap the picture there) and saw that he had a large pneumothorax, a partial collapse of the lung. So we called the surgeons, who placed a chest tube in-between his ribs to re-expand the lung. Later, in one of the happiest moments since graduating medical school one month before, I saw the sunrise over the Charles River. As the others returned that morning around 6:45 a.m., Dave took a couple of washcloths and ran them under the "boiling water" faucet in the sink and handed one to me to put over my face, as barbers do before giving a customer a shave – my consolation for having gotten no sleep. It felt so good.

During sign-in rounds that day, one of the seniors told us about the MICU journal. It was started in 1980 as a way for us to keep track of our experiences as we rotated through that place. I grabbed one of the six volumes off a shelf in the corner of the room and started flipping through. It had some great stories, musings, poetry, and drawings. The first volume was missing its cover; the most recent already included some quotes from the previous day's rounds. The senior explained that by reading the entries from years earlier, some of them by current attendings who were scared residents at the time, we would see that we were part of a shared experience. I took the journal to heart that month and over the next two years, added entries about patients who stood out, about my colleagues' and my experiences, and even newspaper clippings or cartoons. Most of the writing took place late at night; particularly heartfelt entries drew praise and support from the rest of the team the next day. I began to realize how the Journal helped put this strange MICU existence into context by recording the collective experience of a generation of doctors. I then wondered whether it could serve a similar role for patients and their families.

Mikkael A. Sekeres, M.D., M.S.

First Encounters with Death in the MICU

As a medical student, when I was on my surgery rotation, one of our patients died in the middle of the night, in the surgical ICU. It followed a code, one that involved giving a lot of IV fluids, using the cardiac defibrillator ("shocking" a patient), giving high-dose blood pressure medications, epinephrine (adrenaline), and then finally giving up. Everyone left the room except for me and the intern I shadowed for the month. In fact, I'm not sure "shadowed" is a strong enough word. I followed him as if I were attached to him with glue. I slept when he slept, woke with him, ate with him, and went through mood swings with him, which occurred fairly frequently given that he was near the end of his internship year and was pretty toxic – our terminology to describe a combination of depression and anger. At the time I couldn't understand why he was so moody, or why the slightest mishap (a forgotten lab; having to draw blood on a patient; being called to a floor to sign orders) would set him off. Now, we had just been through a code together, and were standing in the room with a dead body. A dead body who had joked around with us on rounds earlier that morning. He turned to me.

"Have you ever been in a room with a body before?"

"Anatomy class. Does that count?"

"Not really. You never saw them alive beforehand. So do you know how to pronounce someone?"

"Listen to their heart (for heart sounds). Shine a light in their eyes (to determine if their pupils respond)."

"Yeah, that's kinda it."

He walked me through it slowly, I think in a way letting the reality of this person's death sink in. I thought about that night as I stood outside Mrs. G's room in the MICU, curtains drawn, family members and friends still surrounding her bed, crying and holding each other. Dave came up to me.

"Are you gonna go in and pronounce her?"

"Yeah." I clearly sounded very uncertain.

"Are you sure? Have you done this before?"

"Oh yeah, I've done it." This time more certain, though by no means convincing.

"All you do is listen with your stethoscope for a couple of minutes for a heartbeat, make sure she's not breathing, shine a light in her eyes, and fill out the death certificate. It's easy." He clapped me on the back.

I went into the room and looked around at the people there, and all I could think of to say was: "I'm sorry. I'm so sorry." They nodded back, a couple of grim half-smiles, a lot of crying. Luckily, one family member, a sister I think, told the others: "The doctor has to examine her now." They stepped away from the bed and stood against the wall, all eyes on me. I hadn't planned this very well beforehand. I figured I would just examine her the same way I had examined her that morning, when she was still alive. But it wasn't that easy. I went to the head of her bed, took out my stethoscope, and placed its diaphragm on her chest while I discreetly eyeballed my watch. And I listened.

Silence.

And listened.

Silence.

I figured time must be up by now and glanced at my watch. Thirty seconds had passed. You've got to be kidding. Thirty seconds??? I glanced at the family. Their eyes were pinned on me. I kept listening.

Silence.

One minute. I was sweating, my back hurt, and this was the longest two minutes of my life. Ninety seconds. They must think I'm crazy by now. They can't be watching me still. I glanced up – they were. Fifteen more seconds. Ten. Five. I stood up, took out my penlight, and opened her eyes. She was cold. Her pupils did not react. With her eyes open, I realized this was not at all like the exam I performed on her that morning. There was no substance to her, no interaction with my movements, my maneuvers. This was all very, very wrong, very un-natural. No signs of breathing. I closed her eyes and faced her family. They thanked me, which I just couldn't believe - for being the one to confirm she was dead. They had the strength to realize, even beyond their own grief, how hard this was for me. Such kindness in the face of sorrow.

Mikkael A. Sekeres, M.D., M.S.

Reflections on Life in the MICU: Control and Order

In the final week of our tour of duty in the MICU, we had one piece of unfinished business. Over the course of the month, we had exchanged messages with the nurses using the computer screen savers located at stations around the MICU. On the whole, pretty innocent stuff: "MICU NURSES RULE!!!!;" "JULY HOUSESTAFF ROCK!!!;" that sort of thing. It was good for everyone's morale, particularly after all the deaths we had witnessed. At some point around the third week of July, though, someone in management decided that the screen savers were unprofessional and demanded they be stopped. They weren't. So the computer techs were called in to lock the screen saver function, so the only message displayed read: "REMEMBER TO WASH YOUR HANDS." Every single terminal in the MICU had the same, boring message. It drove our SAR crazy.

"Remember to wash our hands???!!! How patronizing. Do they think we're busboys?"

Every day during rounds, I'd see his eyes wander to the computer screens during a particularly lengthy, disjointed, post-call intern presentation, and he'd crinkle his forehead and shake his head. You could tell he was simmering, and would blow at any second. He'd re-focus for a while, but then his attention would wander again. Our final day rolled around, and of course Dave and I were on-call for one last time. How fitting to end where we had begun! Morning rounds started as usual, but then the SAR stopped a discussion about management of a patient's ventilator.

"Sekeres!"

"What?" I figured I had forgotten to order a medication or was about to get questioned about pulmonary esoterica.

"I want you to leave rounds and break into those computers and change that damn message. And I don't want you back here until you're successful."

"Really?" I looked to Dave for some clue about whether or not he was joking. Dave shrugged his shoulders. The SAR answered me.

"Sekeres, this may be more important than anything you ever do as a resident. We cannot leave here without restoring order to this place. Our order."

Wow. He sounded like the police chief of Gotham City. I think I just got the Bat Signal. When I was in middle school, personal computers had just hit the market. Our school had TRS-80 computers, and I was part of a "computer club" who would stay after school to do some programming and play games. Now, try using that story as a pick-up line in a bar! At malls, I would stop by Radio Shack stores and play around with one of their display computers, writing simple programs in BASIC. I remember looking up on a couple of occasions and discovering a crowd of people surrounding me, watching in amazement as if I were a savant or some kind of circus freak. Programming was wild, new stuff in the early 1980s! I now realized that this geeky, sheltered part of my life, which I had long ago shed when I substituted contact lenses for my wire-rimmed glasses, was all part of a master plan to prepare me for this moment.

I left rounds and slinked off to a terminal in the corner. There would be no gawking crowds this time. After rounds another intern, Bill, joined me. We worked on it all morning and all afternoon, trying different approaches through both Windows and MS-DOS without much success. Finally, around 5:00 in the evening, we interrupted the computer's boot-up, went in through a back door into MS-DOS, and edited the program that defined the screen saver message. We re-booted the computer, held our breaths, and saw the fruits of our labor:

"MICU NURSES RULE!!!!"

We yipped and hollered and called the team over, and we all caused a huge ruckus. The nurses were thrilled. Immediately, messages went up around the MICU espousing our virtues, the nurses', and making polite suggestions about what the management could do with their clean hands. It brought everyone together, even more so than the flowers we had given the nurses and the cookies they had baked for us, to celebrate the end of our rotation.

Dave and I looked with pride at those screens all night, for once a quiet night in which we got a little sleep. At this point in the rotation, Dave let me answer most of the nurses' questions and manage some of the patients on my own. Without my realizing it fully, I had learned a lot of medicine since orientation. The next day, as we gave morning sign-out to the new MICU team, I once again saw that look of horror on the faces of my fellow interns. The look that says: "Am I going to look that bad after that horrible a night when I'm on call in this place?" I could care less. I was done.

I went to one of the medical floors and "picked-up" my new team of patients – in other words, received a sign-out detailing the medical issues of the new set of patients I would be following for the next month. I almost started laughing when I heard about their medical problems: infection of the toe; an asthma flare; awaiting placement in a nursing home; some heart failure. They were so healthy compared to the patients for whom I had just cared! This would be a piece of cake compared to the MICU.

Mikkael A. Sekeres, M.D., M.S.

CHAPTER ONE:
Introduction to the MICU

Intensive Care Units (ICUs) were created to care for critically ill patients – people who, without modern medical technology and staff, would have a slim chance of surviving. Even despite this "intensive care," about 25% of the patients who enter ICUs in the nation will not leave their hospitals alive. The patients occupying the seventeen beds in the MICU at the MGH are among the sickest in the Northeast, often transferred by ambulance or helicopter ("Medflight") from other hospitals in Massachusetts or other New England states. MGH is a tertiary care, or specialty, hospital, and for many transferred patients it is the place of last resort.

The MICU at the MGH has undergone many changes over the years. At its inception in the 1960s a single ventilator (breathing machine) filled a whole wall in a patient's room. In the late 1970s, the entire unit had the capacity of only two invasive blood pressure monitoring devices (arterial lines, or A-lines), compared to seventeen today. Modern ventilators stand three feet tall and two feet wide, and almost every patient not only has an A-line, but has the information recorded by that line transmitted to monitors at the nurses' station, accompanied by digital message boards throughout the Unit that warn of abnormalities of heart rhythm, blood pressure, or even breathing. Staffing in the MICU includes nurses, who have received specialized additional training in ICU medicine and who care for a maximum of only two patients at a time; respiratory therapists, who are experts at managing ventilators and interpreting the data from those machines; and the attending physicians and residents. In the MICU at the MGH

1

the attending physicians are specialists in pulmonary and critical care medicine, while at other institutions or in other ICUs within the MGH they may specialize in anesthesiology, cardiology, neurology, pediatrics, neonatology, or surgery.

Whether you enter a patient's room in the MICU as a relative, friend, social worker, priest, or member of the hospital staff, you may be overwhelmed by the onslaught of technology. First, there are the IV lines attached to machines that regulate the amount of medication, saline, blood products, or nutrition a patient receives. These machines are clamped to a separate "IV pole" or to poles along the bed corners or along a back bar. At the other end, IV lines enter the patient's veins, either through catheters in his arms or legs or through his neck or chest, the latter called central venous catheters. One type of medication a patient can receive only in an ICU, and only through a central venous catheter, is a high-potency cardiac medication, called a "pressor." This medication is used for patients with extremely low blood pressure, or extremely poor heart function. Next, an A-line, which is placed through a patient's wrist into his radial artery; it measures blood pressure, heart rate, and body temperature. These recordings are displayed on a monitor, somewhere by the patient's bedside. Wires are attached to the patient's chest to record heart rhythms, and to a small device covering one finger or an ear lobe to measure how well the patient is getting oxygen into the blood. These recordings, too, show up on the bedside monitor.

The ventilator is probably the most intimidating piece of equipment in the room. Introduced in 1929, mechanical ventilation came into widespread use in the mid-1950s to replace the "iron lungs" used to support polio victims. Ventilators provide breathing support to patients with lung injuries, either from diseases of recent onset (pneumonia, fluid on the lungs from congestive heart failure, or a blood clot to the lungs) or from chronic, long-standing diseases (e.g., cystic fibrosis, Lou Gehrig's Disease, lung cancer). The machine is attached to a plastic tube that enters the patient's mouth, ending about halfway down his throat. It provides varying amounts of pure oxygen (the air we breathe has 21% oxygen; the machine can provide 100% oxygen) and different amounts of breathing support, from full support (required when the patient cannot even initiate a breath) to partial support (when the ventilator gives an extra "push" once the patient starts a breath). Ideally, a patient will remain on the ventilator for only a short period, a day or two. The longer a patient remains on the ventilator, the more likely the machine itself will start to cause lung injury. While it is needed to maintain adequate oxygen supply in a patient with bad lung disease, the high-dose oxygen the machine provides eventually can damage lung tissue.

The ideal candidate for a stay in the ICU is a patient with a short-term, curable illness: a young person with severe asthma or a bad pneumonia who requires the ventilator for a couple of days until she can breathe on her own again; a man with a bleeding ulcer who needs blood pressure support until his ulcer is repaired; or a woman who, having just suffered a heart attack, needs intensive monitoring to make sure she does not experience a cardiac arrest. Yet, most occupants of ICU beds are frail, elderly people destined to die from chronic diseases but are kept alive by the use of this advanced technology. Physicians wrestle with the power and limits of ventilators, A-lines, monitors, and pressors as much as family members do.

Mikkael A. Sekeres, M.D., M.S.

January 21, 1980

The purpose of this volume is for us to learn from our collective experience. On an individual basis, we know the joys and the horrors of residency training, but often this knowledge is kept to ourselves. A record of what it is we go through will help others avoid the traps of depression, isolation, insecurity, and anger. Anonymous or not, the thrills and spills you provide (both cognitive and affective) are welcome. Enjoy.

(Signed) Ted Stern

June 25, 1995--First Day of Internship

The "deer in the headlights" look is prevalent as we begin this "37-day month" (13 **call days**), thereby defying all lunar or Greco-Roman calendars. On our first day (in the first hour) a patient **VF arrested** in front of us during rounds, and we admitted the official ICU mascot--Mr. L--who is in this book more than many of the house officers. I didn't think I'd be back so soon to say this, but . . . hang on for the ride!

May, 1995

My personal thoughts as we enter week #4 of the MICU:

This morning I awoke feeling **toxic** as all Hell. I roller-bladed into work, stopped at Starbucks for a coffee and oatmeal scone with the stuff on top, and proceeded to MGH with a good attitude. I convinced myself that I have only one week left and I'm going to enjoy it. On sign-in rounds, at 7:30 AM, my intern and I learned of our first admission already awaiting us in the **pit**: A 70-year-old woman with **multiple sclerosis, s/p** an **asystolic arrest**. She was wheeled up to the unit, **mottled, apneic, vented**, and died within the hour. . .A typical MICU experience. Need I say more?

January, 1992

Federal law requires truth in advertising. Dr. S suggests that the **Bigelow 9** name be changed to M.E.C.U--Medical Eternal Care Unit.

Commonly, house officers try to put on an optimistic and happy face. However, more often than not, their optimism is dashed by the realities of critical illness. After weeks-on-end of fighting death, even the most forward-looking young physicians become demoralized and hardened.

August, 1985

Now is as good a time as any to begin to put the month in the ICU in perspective. An appropriate day—with an impending hurricane of devastating proportions approaching our shores from Cape Hatteras. More importantly, it's the morning after call, having gotten a **no hitter**!! With about 6 hours of uninterrupted sleep. Thus, for the first time all month, I'm not in a coma at rounds. So here it goes:

1. The nurses—what a great surprise. Good, no excellent!! relations this year with limited exceptions. Mutual respect, tolerance and shared good/bad times were the order of the day... Actually sad to go.

2. The **visit**—alas every Beaver needs his Wally; every Lassie his Timmy, every **JAR** a **SAR**... Clearly the best and the brightest—all the MGH is supposed to be.

The system—no, I haven't become a milquetoast. The anger is there, it just gets tedious banging your head against the same wall. It seems to me—after 3 years of testing this hypothesis—that telling someone that they don't know shit from a tree is not the best way to convince people of the rectitude of your view. Informing various assholes of their "neutral" qualities seems to have changed nothing. Thus, the system is unlikely to get better, in spite of the "best intentions" of those who run it. The MGH (as distinct from "the system") is indeed a remarkable scene. The house staff give it 100% all the time. Take what you can from the MGH, and when the price gets too dear, cash in the chips and move. There's more to be said, but the hurricane begins.

"Looks like we're in for stormy weather."

P.S. A more appropriate parting line would be:
"With half damp eyes, I stared into the room,
Where my friends and I spent many an afternoon,
Where we together weathered many a storm,
Laughing and singing into the early hours of the morn." Bob Dylan.

Buoyed by the luxury of uninterrupted sleep, the opportunity for reflection arises, but it does not dissipate the entrenched self-criticism, or criticism of the system. Though, like the weather, realities come and go.

May, 1980

I watched "General Hospital" on TV for the first time last week when I had the flu. It's not as dramatic as real life.

August, 1994--7:00 a.m.

I kiss my wife goodbye and enter the mammoth hospital that is slowly and sadly becoming a second home. My first inpatient rotation is in the MICU, overwhelming both on an intellectual and emotional level. This feeling of inadequacy is basically suppressed as I join my JAR on morning rounds, gathering numbers, wondering when that blasted tech is going to **run the bloods** today. Our first patient is a 28-year-old woman with rapidly progressive **respiratory failure**, on **ECMO/CVVH/Pentobarb coma**. The last bit is mind-boggling--we preserved her brain by inducing coma, but we have no idea what will be left if by some miracle she pulls through. The fleeting and false hope of a lung transplant is in the works, but we know it will never happen. If I stop to think about it, I know that woman is going to die, but choose not to think about this fact. Unbelievable technology to keep her alive, hundreds of thousands of dollars, and a hoard of consultants--will it be for naught? Best not to think about it.

11:00 a.m.--Attending Rounds

Cancelled due to an early a.m. admission. K is 17, one week away from starting college, every bit the beautiful, talented teenager we all hope to raise some day. He was found in respiratory distress on the kitchen floor. In the ER, he underwent **CPR** for 45 minutes. He had a massive **pulmonary embolus**, and is now in the unit. Parents and siblings are huddled around him, holding his hand. I fight back my tears.

A third admission is Mr. D, an end-stage **cystic fibrosis** patient who is 3rd on the lung transplant list. His wife used to sleep in the hospital, extremely devoted, calming him during those long nights on **masked ventilation**. However, over the past two weeks, she has started going home for longer stretches each day, perhaps the beginnings of letting go. For now, they pray for a lung transplant.

Lunchtime: Light conversation. The SAR tells stories from his 'pothead' days in high school.

3:00 p.m.: I made small talk with Mr. D's wife as I threaded an **A-line** into her husband. Success!

6:00 p.m.: Sign-out Rounds: Everyone wishes us a quiet night.

9:00 p.m.: I go to get dinner, dispatched by my junior resident, who was **flogging** a **central line** in a new admission with severe **pancreatitis**. He is sick as shit, but hey, it's time to eat! Priority!

7

11:00 p.m.: I admit our 3rd admission, an "easy" one, perfect for my non-expertise. A young man with a **variceal** bleed. Now stable, but sleepy and drunk. He'll survive this madness and go home likely the next day, while my other patients are victims of disease processes not due to any fault of their own. I try not to think about this fact too much.

1:00 a.m.: I place the "finishing" touches on my admission note, when I hear a cry from one of the corner rooms. This is Mr. I, a 50-year-old man with lung destruction due to **IPF**, but thus far has avoided the **tube**, which would represent the beginning of the end. My JAR, tied up with the sick -as -shit pancreatitis dude, leaves me, the scared, tired and inexperienced intern with the rest of the floor. I try giving some anti-anxiety meds, with his respiratory rate of 40. He looks like stool. We avoid **intubating** him. I decide to lie down in an empty room. I lie there for all of 15 seconds when . . .

2:00 a.m.: Mr. D has a seizure. The nurses rush in and begin **bagging** him, but he starts to **aspirate** and needs protection for the sliver of lung function he has left. We intubate him and I call the wife at home, she sleepingly answers. I tell her--gently, of course--about the course of events, that her husband just got intubated. She decides to come in, knowing full well that she may not be able to hear her husband's frail voice again.

2:30 a.m.: Another end-stage **lunger** starts to breathe at 40 breaths per minute. We avoid the tube for now.

3:15 a.m.: My junior is still stuck with the sick pancreatitis dude, so I quickly round on the other patients. An 80-year-old grandfather whose grandson sits with him all night, is in the next room. He'll pull through, having suffered a heart attack. My JAR is in the next room.

The juxtaposition of the recovering grandfather and the two young people--again, too deep a thought to entertain that night.

3:30 AM: I greet Mrs. D and give her a brief hug as she is in tears.

4:00--4:45 AM: The sick pancreatitis dude has an **asystolic arrest** and dies. He only lasted 7 hours at MGH after his transfer.

4:45 AM: Mr. I, still breathing at a rate of 40 breaths per minute, gets intubated.

6:00 AM: Gathering **numbers** for sign-in rounds. Family is still gathered around K's bed, continuing their vigil.

7:00 AM: Residents arrive to find our uneaten dinners on the table. They offer their condolences for our terrible night and lack of sleep. We begin pre-rounds again.

9:00 AM: Mr. D goes into **cardiac arrest**. We take turns compressing his chest. He comes back briefly. His wife, meanwhile, is crying by the nurses' station.

11:00 AM: Mr. D dies. We pull off our gloves in shock, while the nurses clean him up before transporting him to the morgue and the senior resident goes to inform his wife.

2:00 PM: I leave post-call through the revolving doors, squinting in the bright sun. I take note of the perfect summer breeze and look forward to kissing my wife once again.

There are times when life in the MICU is more dramatic than what is portrayed on television. Contrasts amplify the drama: youth and age,

inexperience and experience, sickness and health, dying patients and liv-
ing families, clear thinking and confusion. To function in this setting, you
often have to check your emotions at the door. In doing so, you shift your
sympathies: the team expressed condolences to the intern and junior, not
to the grieving families.

June, 1994

Signing off from my stint on the Bigelow 9 MICU. List for the new arrivals:
Don't panic.
It's not your fault these people are sick.
Don't tweak the nurses.
Don't be tweaked by the nurses.
If say, for example, a blind diabetic with renal failure and morphine addiction is admitted and she wants her "fix," just remember that the MICU is no place to get the patient to kick her habits and really, you need to sleep.
Wash your hands often.
Good luck, and thanks to the team.

December, 1992

A JAR, giving an intern, a word of wisdom on the rigors of the ICU.
JAR: "One last word of wisdom before we keep signing out: Take care of yourself mentally and physically."
Intern: Pauses, doodles on his sign-out paper.
JAR: "Did you write that down?"

July, 1985

Working with a new intern at the beginning of the year is not unlike having a child. I suppose. The first day you go through all the routine idiosyncrasies of the MGH -- where to get blood sent, how to get **blood gas** results, where to request **films**, and then slowly the interns take on more and more responsibility and begin as they should to run the unit. More than once I've been surprised and pleased at **pup rounds** to hear what they've done. There does seem to be a delicate balance between watching out or watching over them and leaving them alone enough for them to do their work and learn from it. It's almost sad that after 4 weeks I almost felt superfluous in the ICU at afternoon pup rounds since I've been absorbed in the **White 8** business. Contrast that feeling to the sense of being indispensable on the first day.

Of course, that's how the year progresses. And that's part of the transition between being an intern and being a junior....

Leafing through volume 3 of "**The Red Book**" in which I have made most of the entries, one would think that the unit is a fun place to work—a laugh a minute. It is. But it's much more than that. But to understand you have to be there.

Rules for the uninitiated come in many forms. Some are practical, some humorous, some cynical or sadistic. Whichever it is, the preparation is intended to help us cope with what lies ahead.

March, 1990

Yes, here it is. The fourth exciting volume of the MGH house staff "**red book**." The third volume ran out 3 months ago and when I came to write my useless thoughts here found there were no pages left. So I took Ted Stern's job upon myself (MGH **H.O.**'s like to take initiative) and bought volume 4 this week. Why the color blue? Well the last two volumes of the "red book" were black, often confusing interns. So I figured why not add to the confusion by making the red book blue. Not to mention that blue is my favorite color and I have this thing for women with blue eyes.

So once again, all are invited to write in this book with your name or anonymously if you prefer. Reflections, stories, funny situations from rounds, comments about the place or this program are all fair game. Of course, more serious concerns and thoughts about life, residency, or patient care are also welcome.

And don't forget that when life in the unit starts getting you down, the best thing to do is quickly escape to the conference room, pick up an old copy of the red book and read about the trials and tribulations of the overworked, underpaid and metabolically completely unstable MGH medical house staff.

November, 1997

Already day #6 and I haven't written in the book. Lots of things to write (most pretty funny) but it's 5:45 PM and expressing myself here would be more of a **flog** than anything else.

September, 1998

MICU motto: "First, don't do much harm."

A derivative of a passage from the Hippocratic Oath: "First - Do no harm."

May, 1993

Our SAR, on making about 7 patients **DNR** today, as we near the end of the month: "I feel like the end of a Clint Eastwood movie--"bang, bang, bang" and everyone's dead."

May, 1986

The ICU really isn't a bad place when you aren't working here...

Februrary, 1981

Yes, the ICU can be the ultimate in **iatrogenesis**, the road to **Allen Street**, but it can just as rapidly be the opposite. The 1 in 10 cure. The room 3 survivor....sees you in clinic doing well. The **septic, acidotic, hypoxic, hypotensive, hypothermic**, hypo-this, hyper-that, survivor who shakes your hand as he leaves the hospital at the front door. The man you **cardioverted** 20 times in one evening and **CPR**'d until your arms hurt who survives to say thanks. The **train wreck** transfer from surgery who you **buff** and send back. It is here in the good old ICU where you really first begin to feel that we just have something to offer. This is where it's at—I feel good.

Each of the above entries could have been written by the same person. Highs and lows occur often without a predictable cycle, changing from hour to hour, and incident to incident. Interesting that the need to write in the book outweighed the intent to keep emotions to oneself.

August, 1993

These are the best of times, the worst of times. . . there are 4 patients in the MICU; including the attending, that's a housestaff to patient ratio of 2 to 1. The calm before the storm, or a going-out-of-business sale? We wait. . .

October, 1998

Our SAR, (to the **RN** in Ms. V's room): "Hey, Tom, what's the good word?"
Tom: "Where . . . Here?!"

February 23, 1999--4:00 AM--

The last night on Bigelow 9 is passing with a whimper--one easy admission, worked up entirely by a **sub-intern**, everyone else is **meta-stable** (our great MICU word). I sacrifice what little time I have for sleep to make what will be the final entry in this conference room. I cannot summarize the immense past sentiment of our collective house staff with any sort of gestures. I only regret that the only bed to sleep in is taken by my intern while I sit here writing this entry. Finally, a MICU with enough call-room beds--with any call-room at all. To all past house staff who have spent countless sleepless nights here--or slept in a cardiac chair, or on the floor in the conference room, or even on the **Allen Street table**, here is a salute to all the **cheeching**, teaching and finally, unbelievable and extraordinary patient care that has taken place on this unit.

After 22 years, on February 23, 1999, the MICU moved to a new and more technologically sophisticated space in the hospital. The former MICU residence, whence these entries come, contained no room in which residents could sleep – as space within the hospital became tight, these rooms were eliminated. Instead, residents on-call slept wherever they could - in empty patient rooms, in chairs, even on the morgue stretcher. In such a unit, it is easy to imagine why nobody would expect a house officer to sleep…

January, 1984

Tonight we admitted a man, an architect who had a **VF arrest** at a conference in Boston, away from his family who are in Arizona. They can't come because it's snowing and the airport's closed. He's **decorticate**.

They feel afraid and helpless. It's pretty sad. This unit can be full of sadness like that. That's part of the intensity of it.

March, 1981

In overview, the Bigelow ICU is a place filled with broken bodies, expensive machinery, stressed and tired doctors, overworked nurses, and frightened families all trying in their varied ways to cope with fear, death, and personal feelings. It's a draining experience and one in which the forest itself often obscures the trees (i.e., the patients). It's much easier to check the **wedge, I/O's**, and blood pressure than to spend the time talking to a 45-year-old about his sub-massive **MI**. The forest of numbness and paperwork so often insulates us from the patients and their grieving/frightened families and, in doing so, helps "protect" us from sharing similar experiences. Too much isolation, however, makes us technocrats and not physicians. The ICU really is a crucible into which we place our medical knowledge, emotions, humor, anxieties, and idiosyncrasies and, via a refining process, emerge somewhat changed individuals. Generalizing the experience is useless for it must be different for each individual.

June, 1996

Nothing funny tonight on this first night on call. What is on my mind is just how much I've changed since my month here 3 years ago as a student. Then, I was taken by the complexity of the patients, the constant tinkering, adjustment and perfecting of care, and the fun we had in the midst of death/despair/frustration. Still, my reaction is very different. We have a great team; I can already tell we're going to have a lot of fun this month. But what I can't stop thinking about as I adjust the patient's **vent** or replete someone's potassium, or pronounce someone dead is how much more we could be doing for other, less sick, people, with the same amount of time, effort, and mental energy.

We spend a lot of time on these patients but the rewards are few, and the great saves come, at best, 3 or 4 times per month. Is it all worth it? But these are just thoughts going through my head tonight. Actually, I love this place. It's always fun, sometimes frustrating, but sometimes also, exhilarating. The way I look at things, a good **code**, (crisis, whatever) is like savoring a bottle of fine wine. It's definitely something to go over and over again, even if it leaves you with a headache in the morning.

May, 1997

Dr. K, a JAR, after his last traumatic night on call, says during sign-in: "Don't send me out there!"

Sometimes, like battle-worn foot soldiers in a foreign land, residents plead not to be sent back to the fray.

October, 1991

Morning rounds were ugly today: The Intern and JAR on Team 1 complaining that once again the intern and JAR on Team 2 had another golden night with only one admission; Team 2 complaining that Team 3 weren't doing their jobs of finding the nurses and **books for rounds**, etc. There were also three deaths this week so far. Deep down we are all still friends—it's just been a long month, and we are finally seeing the light at the end. Until then tensions will continue to wax and wane.

September, 1997

I'm back on Medicine after a year on **Neuro**. It's hard to believe that I've only spent a total of two months here--2 weeks as a pre-lim **PGY1**, 4 weeks as a JAR, and now, 2 weeks as a SAR. All the staff seem so happy to see me--"You again?!" "Aren't you Neuro?!" It's been great to be back, but I do feel like an old-timer, and I couldn't resist the temptation to pour myself out in the book. This unit is undoubtedly one of the greatest places in the hospital to work -- with the "best" cases, nursing, respiratory and house staff teams--but remains as humbling and depressing as ever. Even the Neuro ICU is more uplifting. . .

I've been here a lot as the neuro consult, but it's much harder being on the team itself, feeling emotionally invested in the patients, and then seeing them go down the tubes. On the Neuro Service, they come in **stroked-out**, we often never know them as people. Neurologic disease is unfortunately frustrating therapeutically and prognostically, but it's so much worse here in the setting of **multi-system organ failures**. I'm supposed to be an asset to the team as a neuro "expert;" instead, I leave feeling depressed and defeated--I can't offer what they really want--a good outcome.

-R

September, 1997

To R,

Don't feel defeated. We'll miss the knowledge and experience you brought to the team. We never would have been able to respond as smoothly to the neuro crises if you weren't "a room away." Thanks for all your help and support.

Surrounded by a critical mass of illness, with uncertain and, at times, devastating outcomes, it is no wonder that intra-squad squabblings smolder and sometimes boil over. The intensity of the work brings people together. Like a family, tempers often erupt, later to be counterbalanced by support, dependence, and mutual respect.

May, 1985

Last ICU day note.

I feel like I'm being let out of prison. It's a combination of relief, exhilaration, and sense of having passed through something difficult. I'm going to miss the unit, though. I'll miss morning rounds, with the SAR rushing us along, with the discussions of **acid-base disorders** on renal patients of little clinical significance, I'll miss Mr. T, whose only event each day is how long he **weaned** and whether he got his **Fleets enema**.

I'll miss **running the list** every 4 hours. I'll miss the procedures—the thrill of getting spurting blood back from an **A-line**—or the frustration and feeling of incompetence when I have trouble putting one in.

The unit has a life all its own. All of us—the interns, residents, nurses, patients—all come and go. But the unit lives on. And we get to be part of it. For a time.

October, 1990

After almost a year and a half at the MGH, one wouldn't expect to be surprised too much at the "goings-on." But this has been an extraordinary month. 31 days of wild and wooly, non-stop action in the Bigelow ICU, and I was happy, proud, sad, frustrated to be a part of the commotion...things hardly settled down after the first day but our team did develop a rhythm, a harmony of sorts, and we began to observe a meaningful quality in this factory of human lives intertwined with machinery and technology. During this production some patients lived, some patients died, and some patients simply stayed. None were forgotten. Fortunately, our team had no illusions about saving the dead, and for those without life left we let go, gently. The nurses and staff were wonderful...our team had fun too and was not without boisterous moments, crazy times. We came to truly enjoy one another's company amidst the turmoil. Of course, sign out after 9 p.m. became a bit tiresome.

The month ended with a fire in the basement of the MGH. We moved many patients and were left with a skeleton crew of 10 patients, the least (by far) all month. It was a fitting end to an incredible month, one which I will remember for many, many years.

April, 1994

After a long, sleepless night on call, the intern notices that morning has arrived: "I can see the sun glinting off the **vent**."
JAR: "Oh, that is so sad."

Even when someone tries to be sensitive, poetic, and supportive, another person is always there to burst the bubble and bring him or her back to earth.

June, 1993

What a way to end your residency, finishing as captain of the **Death Star**, and ending the "book." This place, like residency, should only be done once. It is an experience that can only truly be understood by those who have had similar times. If I had to do it all over again, I'd do it in an instant. The experience was superb. I couldn't imagine packing the highs and lows of intellectual and emotional success and strain any other way. . . . I leave with tremendous sentiments of nostalgia and satisfaction for a time of my life well worth having."

January, 1998

Welcome, kind sir to the MICU.
It's my special job to inflict you.
With all sorts of pain
To your Art'ries and veins
'Til there's no place left to stick you.

When critically ill patients are treated in the MICU, it is essential for physicians to gain access to the vascular anatomy, that is, the arteries and veins. Doctors need access to the arteries for invasive monitoring of blood pressure, heart rate, and oxygenation (as opposed to a blood pressure cuff, which would be "non-invasive"). Access to the arteries also allows for frequent, painless blood draws and interventions (as in a cardiac assist device). To place an arterial (or "A-line") into an artery, a resident first washes the patient's wrist with betadine soap, and then injects lidocaine (or Novacaine) into the wrist, to make it numb. Then, she feels for a pulse (indicating the location of the artery, which does not push outward from the skin like some veins) and aims a needle with a catheter sheath (like a sleeve over an arm) into the lumen (or inside tunnel) of the artery. When she sees a pulsing return of blood through the outside end of the needle, she removes it, leaving the blunt sheath in the artery. Then, she threads a thin wire through the sheath into the artery lumen and advances the sheath over the wire farther into the artery, to secure it better. This is known as the "Seldinger" technique. Finally, she removes the wire, leaving the sheath deeply imbedded in the artery, and sews the sheath to the skin using thin thread, to secure it even better. The catheter then is attached to monitoring equipment.

December, 1994

Our SAR regarding: Mr. B, with overwhelming **sepsis**, **pancreatitis**, and a **Ph of 6.9**, who is making some progress: "If he makes it, we're going to the supermarket, getting a piece of chicken, hooking it up to a **vent, pressors**, and 6 antibiotics and bringing it back to life."

Critical illness often causes many organs to fail simultaneously. At times it is hard to imagine that a person with such multi-organ failure will survive.

May, 1993

Once they're **intubated**, paralyzed and sedated, it's like a videogame."

When a person loses the ability to communicate, is unresponsive to questions, and technology is rampant, physicians may forget they are caring for a human being, or depersonalize the patient as a reaction to his/her profound illness.

November, 1993

During rounds, our attending philosophizes: "This is the ICU. . . If we're wrong, we **intubate**."

December, 1993

SAR: "Let's try the **VA wean**."
Team: "What's that?"
SAR: "Just lighten him up. . . untie his hands, and when he's ready, he'll yank the **tube**."

The Veterans Administration system of medical care has been burdened with an unfair stereotype of poor care. In conjunction with this notion, the Vets exposed to this care are believed able to survive any procedure, any disease, any trial.

April, 1992

Our attending, commenting about micro-managing vented patients who are stable: "Imagine a politically-volatile Caribbean island, you're at the airport, guns are pointing at everyone, and someone says: "No one moves, no one gets hurt.""

May, 1998

The visiting pulmonologist from Brazil thought the greatest idea he could bring back to his Intensive Care Unit after a visit with us was a **rectal bag**.

October, 1993

The MICU version of "Indecent Proposal," a popular movie with Robert Redford and Demi Moore.

About the patient with a large **rectal tube** with retained loose stool:

JAR #1: "How much money would it take to get you to take one big suck on the end of that tube?"

JAR #2: "About $5,000."

JAR #1: (Aghast!): "I wouldn't do it for any less than $500,000."

June, 1996

Well, it's my last night as an intern here. I've made several observations here in the unit, only some of which are of any importance. I feel there's an observation that's important to share with others. Unfortunately, my audience will be limited by colloquial differences. I've noticed that when interns present patients on rounds, and bend over the **blue books** to read off patient data, they kind of remind me of somebody at their *bar or bat mitzvah*. Think about it.

When faced with the horror of individuals losing control of their bodily functions, absurd associations arise; the more absurd, the more palatable the situation becomes by comparison. Not all associations or analogies are grotesque. But they still provide a degree of comfort and distance.

February, 1990

An incredible day in the ICU! A transformer blew in the sub-basement and filled the stairways with smoke. This prompted a 1-minute interruption in power and the team/nurses **bagging** patients until auxiliary power kicked in. Furthermore with smoke we evacuated seven patients with full transfer orders and transfer notes in a matter of 1 hour. After a.m. rounds, one JAR comments how much work was achieved and that usually it would take all day to transfer so many patients. Another JAR stated, "Yeah! We really worked hard!" Our SAR rhetorically came back, "Oh yeah, anyone can work that fast when you have a fire under you!"

December, 1998

Dr. O, a JAR, opening her fortune cookie, post-call after a devastating night with 6 admissions and 2 deaths:
"You should be of more tenderness and less aggressiveness."

July, 1996

The Ultimate MICU **Dispo**:
A 72-year-old man who was traveling on a cruise ship from Nova Scotia to New York, unfortunately became sick near the Boston Harbor and after docking, was rushed to Mass. General, only to find himself in the Bigelow 9 ICU with **endocarditis**, **meningitis**, and a **splenic abscess**. Well, he was quite discontent and insisted on returning home to Las Vegas.

Well, being the obedient SAR, I obeyed his wishes, making sure he was aware of the risks of such a request.

At 8:00 PM, a flight crew arrived to take him to a Lear jet to fly him back to Las Vegas from Boston. I don't know if he made it, but I do know that it cost him $12,000.00.

You pay your money and you take your chances.

October, 1995

The duration of the moratorium on house officers sleeping in patients' beds following a death, was the topic of discussion. The consensus was 24--48 hours, the actual length of time found to be dependent on their grotesqueness and canine-ness of the circumstances, i.e., whether it was merely a dog show, or a dog/pony show. Dr. F took issue with the majority opinion: "I don't care. I'll sleep in the bed with the corpse."

As the MICU lacked a residents' call room, house officers slept in empty patients' beds – sometimes, newly-empty.

May, 1994

Our SAR, feeling down about the fact that all our **players** are dying, states: "I think I'll go to the more cheery side of the MICU." (Where we have only two patients expected to die in the next 12 hours).
HMS: "The what?"
SAR: "The more cheery side."
HMS: "Oh, I swear to God, I thought she said the mortuary side" . . .

April, 1994

"April is the cruelest month." --T.S. Eliot

April, 1990

As a final thought for this month: "The horror, the horror."—Joseph Conrad, Heart of Darkness.

November, 1993

Just passed the halfway point--the unit has ballooned from 4 quasi-stable patients to a full house of 16 **players**. Our SAR walks into morning rounds stating, "Welcome to my nightmare. . ." You know that when Alice Cooper is quoted on rounds, all is not well.

January, 1980

Well, I don't feel alone tonight, but there is a certain half hollow emptiness. A half-ache rising, falling. Self-confident balloon let loose and whizzing whooooshh across the room. Lights blinking off an on, monitors rotating. Bleep, whoosh, bleep, whoosh. All along the watch tower with respirators instead of phase shifters, Ravel piano concerto in G with monitor alarm piccolos. Oh, how I long for the second movement, the sunshine of tomorrow afternoon's lazy flute over waterfall piano background. Ah, Ravel. Soft and sweet honeydew breath of afternoon rest. And then the third movement, sharp knife-like, like the call to arms, code beeper blaring. Night, all, don't let the bedbugs bite.

Wow.

January, 1980

Certainly a quiet night in the unit. Is this a car wash, wax and **buff**? Amazing how the local lingo creeps into your consciousness until it posses your vernacular being. Ah, the luxury of superfluous language and praise. To use many words and say nothing. To bellow forth like a balloon around the world in 80 days. Zip, flash, dash, crash. Well, it's obvious that the **'tern** is toxic. His **granulations** have the sweet edge. **Toxicology screen** revealed a serum porcelain of 98 and he was started on ivory snow **PR**. I can't wipe white off my mind. White, I wash, coats, jackets, socks, purses, lights. Well, I guess I'll go to sleep. Ah.

Stream of consciousness notwithstanding, can you imagine being cared for by this intern?

June, 1987

Although only completing my junior year, this is also my last night in the ICU. I have chosen not to run the ICU as a senior resident. Why! For those of you who have not done the unit you will see; for those of you who have you know the answer.

There are only so many ways **coronary artery disease** can present and we've seen them all. The learning curve in the ICU peaked long ago. Watching people die with big time **Chi-Chi** is neither educational, nor fun, nor particularly humane. Whoever invented the ICU should see some of the patients we have here. With reference to the atom bomb, Einstein said, "With the development of the bomb, everything has changed save our mode of thinking, and thus we drift perilously." I propose with the invention of the ICU we also need to change our way of thinking. Just because we have the capacity to prolong life in elderly people doesn't mean we have to and yet we do; every day in this place we prolong suffering at little benefit. Bring back the house call and a hold of the hand.

Final score—buried hundreds; saved one or two; cured zero; **flog** on, comrades!

August, 1992

Our SAR, on reviewing the current list of MICU patients for survival potential: "We have a unit of toast."

The death toll for the month is already up to 12, many of whom probably should have been allowed to die before ever coming here.

Just once in a while, it would be nice to treat someone who was sick, but had a decent long-term prognosis. We have had our surprises. . . but our efforts have made very few people become long-term better. Did they live because of us or in spite of us? Did they die because of us, or in spite of us? How should I know? I just work here. . .

February 14, 1997

At this halfway point through the rotation, I paused briefly with an interlude a bit happier than our prior entries. A very strange Valentine's Day, full of our usual mix of hard work and humor, then everyone leaves and the overnight folk begin the task of admitting new patients, putting out fires until, as I put it, the cavalry returns at 7:15 the next morning.

We joked last week that our unit was full of young people--a wonderful statistic of only 3 persons over 60--but the octogenarians had come in numbers. Tonight, we received two elderly women, both with **congestive heart failure**, and began a process of **cheeching** them as we worked them up. Instead of young persons with **sepsis** or sick ones with HIV or cancer, but a fighting shot at life, we run through problem lists a mile long that all begin to sound the same. In the meantime, I'm forced to ignore the rest of the unit, watching the young children come in and out of the room with their 42-year-old mother who just had a large heart attack, or the older children, attempting to look strong as their mother lies dying of cancer and sick with pneumonia. My heart spasms a bit. I run back and forth like a chicken with its head cut off, too much to do, so little time. In all the levity and perversities of our time here, the entire human spectrum can be felt and observed, experienced and lived in, everything from that painful meeting to a pronouncement of death, a not so gentle prod of our seniors to a bite of bagel in the morning, to the sound of my child drifting off to silent sleep, this has been my week. . .

March, 1986

I think our national medical community has its priorities reversed vis-a-vis proper use of medical resources. Here in the ICU we spend hundreds of thousands to millions to keep barely living bodies alive—so that patients and their families can suffer longer. Meanwhile, children die of diarrhea, teenagers continue to smoke, and millions cannot get access to basic medical care—e.g., routine physicals, preventive medicine, outpatient management of diabetes, **hypertension**. Sure, it's much more dramatic to put in a **PA-line** than it is to give a flu vaccine or encourage a patient to quit smoking: to adjust a **pacer** in a patient who was baseline **asystole** or **V-tach** than to check cholesterols and try to adjust them. But which of these modalities benefits more people with lower morbidity. Maybe our health care bill would be more affordable and the public would have more faith in us if we eliminated super critical care, stopped this absurd denial of death and returned to medicine's most basic objectives: alleviation of suffering (not causing it, as we often do in the ICU to both patients and their families) prolongation of life—when there is life to prolong, and the advancement of knowledge.

November, 1994

After a month in this ICU, I am now forced to condemn it as an embarrassment to a modern ethical society. Designed as a vehicle for aggressive therapy for otherwise healthy individuals with acute and potentially reversible medical problems, it has become instead a long-term care facility for individuals permanently incapable of contributing to or deriving enjoyment from the life and community outside. It is an engine of false hope, misperceptions and overall moral negligence. We, as its captains, are universally guilty of prolonging the suffering of those unable to comprehend the complete extent of their decisions, while consuming the resources entrusted to us by society as a whole.

"Doing more" remains the path of least resistance--doing less ought to be the challenge to face up to. We inflict harm in the guise of treatment. As an alternative, perhaps we might devote more effort to overall treatment goals. Place ourselves in the patient's position--we know what the right thing to do is--we need to explain to the families that we understand, and give them permission to draw back. We abuse our power by doing otherwise. Lastly, we might work on physicians to avoid letting our patients get to this point. Few of the millions of people we meet truly want all that is done here. How often do these people change their minds while unable to communicate--how many hate us for what we do?

October, 1996

In an exchange that captures the real MICU: Patient A, a blind, diabetic, **gastroparetic**, renal transplant recipient, who was formerly/formally completely **DNR** (before we **intubated** her and **cheeched** her for a week), responds on rounds, post-**extubation**, to the query "How are you,"

"You sadists. . ."

And we basked in the glow of a job well done.

February, 1995

I have now finished my MICU days. Each time I returned, I liked the place more--I'm not certain what that means. My first two weeks as an intern were mostly miserable, writing long, detailed notes on all the patients while on call--this generally taking up the whole call day. Writing notes and not doing many admissions. The second two weeks as an intern were better, and as a junior, there was a certain sense of confidence, and a better awareness of what was going on. It is probably my four weeks as a senior that I'll remember most. Dealing with the families can be sometimes enjoyable, but often frustrating. You really wonder sometimes what we're doing up here--spending, in some cases, so much time and so many resources on patients whose prognosis is grim. We did, however, learn from one patient--a patient we never expected to make it out--**hepatic coma, peritonitis**, who was started on dialysis. But the family assured us she had made it before, and well she did. But will the family now have unrealistic expectations for further episodes? On the other hand, there were some young patients whom you get a great sense of satisfaction taking care of--ideal MICU patients. A 20-year-old, **intubated** with influenza A, a 25-year-old, intubated with asthma. People who we give full supports to and expect to live normal lives. Oh well, I'll never forget my Bigelow 9 days--I sure have learned a lot from them.

September, 1998

Reflections on a Stellar Month:

My second trip to the MICU has been entirely different, yet equally enjoyable to my first visit. My first rotation as an intern in February of 1996, was memorable for my disbelief over the amount of knowledge I have to master. I was enthralled by the new experience of being a doctor and meeting all my talented peers. This visit, I've been a more involved member of the team. . . and "the team" has made the month one to remember. We have not enjoyed a month of glorious saves, but instead, have poked and prodded a group of patients who were on their way to dying, or tried for weeks to pull someone through, only to fail frustratingly.

What has made this month wonderful has been the interaction of the MICU team; we've had a great month of hilarious sign-outs and sarcastic rounds to help us get through the patients we were "**cheeching**." . . .

I look forward to remembering this month and to telling stories about the team, the jokes and the jokers, we took care of. I'll miss the nurses, the respiratory techs, the clerks, and even a patient or two, but I won't miss any more sleep!

January, 1980

Tonight, thinking about summing up, I flipped through my **cards** from these 30 days. And the conclusion is so evident I'm mystified I (we) ever delude myself (ourselves) into thinking it might be otherwise—75% of the patients we admitted in the last month either had end-stage disease before admission or fell to that **prognosis** soon after admission. Some time way back in the latter half of my internship, I gave up the idea of saving lives and became more comfortable with the idea of managing illness to limit dis-ease. But in the ICU we really aren't even able to do that very much since almost all the definitive maneuvers have already been made or are not any longer an option. As a result, what we do for ourselves and what we do for patients are really two distinct things. For ourselves we manage to learn a great deal about the mechanics of medical care for desperately sick people. For patients and, more importantly, for families, I'm beginning to think what we do is simply provide a dramatic, even gruesome ritual of dying. It seems we fend off death for hours, days, or weeks in an elaborate, mystifying, labored dance so that all concerned can get used to the impending death. Grieving is not easy to learn, hardest of all in sudden, unexpected death. So we do as much as seems reasonable to keep Charon's boat on shore for a few hours and to let everyone have a last glimpse, partly of themselves, partly of the one dying. That's what strikes me most right now....

Caring for patients in the ICU raises issues about aggressive and expensive health care; it is often ambivalent, and disturbing. A lack of definitive answers, guidance, and policies contributes to the distress experienced by house officers.

May, 1994

The best part of the house officer experience is the privilege to work with others - nurses, interns, residents, social workers, faculty and so on. Lending a hand, pitching in together. Cracking jokes as a group - one line spawning yet another one-liner. Sharing the serious moments. Being there when someone's depressed. Occasionally feeling a hand on your shoulder. Sharing moments of success, wonderment, bafflement, unhappiness. Internship isn't so much taking care of patients for me as trying to take care of the friends I've made here. God, this is strange to say but true. Patients are so much less real right now. It's the inner lives of others that compel my care almost as much, sometimes more, than the lives of the patients here. It's an intensive form of care. Reading between the lines in what someone's saying. Seeing the quick flicker of an unvoiced thought pass across an otherwise composed face. Trying to figure out what next thing you can do to make someone feel better and responding to that unvoiced need. Please let's remember that our inner lives deserve intensive care and be good to each other. The pain and anguish we experience is no less real than that of our patients. We can't monitor it with **PA-lines** and seldom will we be congratulated for our diagnostic prowess but the therapeutic results can be most gratifying. Thanks and please forgive the length and terrible syntax. Sleepily.

CHAPTER TWO:

The Code Call

A code call, or "Code Blue," is called on a hospital's overhead paging system on television, in a movie, or in real life, and hordes of doctors, nurses, respiratory therapists, pharmacists, and aides go running into a patient's room. Someone starts shouting orders, tensions are high, it all seems incredibly dramatic. Why would somebody call a code, precipitating this maelstrom of activity, and what is all the fuss about?

A code call can be thought of as calling 911 within a hospital. Somebody, usually a nurse or nurse's aide, sometimes a physician or med student, or even an environmental services worker, discovers a patient unresponsive, and that person needs help FAST! It may be that the patient is in a deep sleep from medication, but more worrisome causes of unresponsiveness include seizure, cessation of breathing, or cessation of heart function (called respiratory arrest or cardiac arrest, respectively). At Mass General, once a code is called, a special team of residents who carry code pagers run to the patient's room from all over the hospital, and begin efforts to resuscitate the patient.

The process of resuscitation (cardiopulmonary resuscitation, or CPR) follows a certain order, delineated by the American Heart Association in its Basic Life Support (BLS) and Advanced Cardiac Life Support (ACLS) algorithms. Every physician and nurse in the hospital is certified in either BLS or BLS and ACLS, and must be recertified every two years. The first principles of resuscitation follow the mnemonic "ABC": establish an Airway, check to see that the patient is Breathing, and ensure that the patient has a Circulation. If the patient does not have a pulse, chest compressions are started. Why the rush to the

33

patient's room? Studies have shown that if these principles of CPR are not initiated within the first thirty seconds following a cardiac arrest, the patient's chances of survival plummet.

One of the senior medical residents, called the "Senior-On-for-the-House," calls the shots in the room. After arriving, usually out-of-breath (not much chance to exercise as a resident!) he or she will ask for a brief history of the patient, that may or may not sway future management. For example, if the patient is in the hospital with a heart attack, the period of unresponsiveness is more likely to have been caused by an abnormal heart rhythm. If the patient has just received a hip or knee replacement, a blood clot to the lungs rises as a possibility. The senior then dictates who will perform chest compressions (usually a med student or intern, with frequent relief – it's incredibly tiring work!), who will draw blood for labs (usually an intern), who will place large IV lines for rapid blood or fluid replacement (usually a junior or senior resident), and who will intubate the patient, administer shocks with the cardiac defibrillator (the "paddles,") and interpret the EKG strips (again, usually a junior or senior). Once the patient is "brought back," (can maintain a blood pressure and normal heart rhythm), he or she is moved to an ICU (if not already in one) for close monitoring.

But what if the patient does not survive? Several studies in the 1980s reviewed in-hospital CPR and found that fewer than half the patients upon whom CPR is initiated are "brought back," and only 10-15% survive to leave the hospital. These are low numbers, though admittedly they occur in people who have underlying illness. Otherwise, why would they be in the hospital? The patients who died tended to be older, to have other diseases (e.g., cancer, kidney failure, pneumonia), and to have received prolonged resuscitation efforts. These are the patients you hope have advance directives, or a "code status," dictating that in the event of a period of unresponsiveness, they not undergo CPR.

Then, when do you decide that you have been resuscitating someone for too long, and that maybe your and everyone else's effort are in vain? After all, if you bring a patient back after an hour of CPR, that person has an abysmal chance of being intact mentally, and then may linger for days in an ICU while his or her family suffers through an undignified death. And yet…there was one woman for whom I led the code as a senior who kept coming back briefly in-between prolonged periods of deterioration. We decided to try one more medication before calling it quits, because we had been at it for forty-five minutes. Well, as it happened the drug worked (or, more likely, she just recovered on her own), and we sent her to the ICU, shaking our heads at her prognosis. I received a page the next day from the MICU, telling me she had woken up and hugged her family. I went to see her and she waved at me from her bed – unbelievable! She was my 10-15%. For every one of her, I sent eight others to the MICU who would die eventually. When do you "call" (end) the code? There is no answer. At a certain point, I think you just realize that you are interfering with the natural course of events.

Mikkael Sekeres, M.D., M.S.

February, 1983

It's over. No more ICU as an intern. Next time I come back, I spend the night in the sack while the **'tern** writes those G-D unit notes. Last night on, I'm ready to go to bed at 1 a.m., unit notes written because the people weren't sick, and after 35 days you can write a lousy, shitty, unit note in 20 minutes or less, whereas it took 40 minutes to write a shitty unit note when you started the rotation. Getting back to story line, 1 a.m. and I'm ready to go to bed. One should never be ready to go to bed in the ICU—you'll always be disappointed. Anyway, I'm on my way to the **EW** to pick up a patient when there's a **code** on Bigelow 9. Get up there and find Dr. G trying to intubate an unfortunate **asthmatic** who is as blue as this ink—I keep thinking—he's blue enough to go to the ICU—I keep hoping he's going to be too blue to go anywhere. Probably a nice man with a caring wife and concerned children, but I don't want that **SOB** to make it because I've already got one EW patient whose going to keep me up 2 more hours—I don't need an **intubated, cardioverted**, SOB to take up a bed in my unit....I don't want the asthmatic SOB to live if it means I don't sleep—I don't want the EW patient to live if it means I don't sleep. I just want to sleep. And I know I'm not going to get any sleep—no point in being pissed, but I am anyway. Get to the EW (the blue cardioverted, asthmatic dies. Now how do you feel? You wanted him dead.) and the other patient is one of the best you've seen yet. 70-year-old with **CAD**, **CHF**, **CABG x 3**, **CVA**, dementia, pneumonia, and **respiratory arrest**.

What half-wit **resuscitated** this man—and what half-wit is going to spend the rest of the night keeping him alive? So, I'm out of bed, not sleeping, not dreaming, getting angrier and angrier because the common sense humane intelligence that bills **pneumococcal pneumonia** as the "old man's friend" doesn't exist anymore. And I'm powerless to change that—I can't let this man die—I have to **flog** this **gome**. That's what the ICU team is all about—flogging gomes. The intern doesn't run the ICU, come to think of it. The ICU—the concept, the medical technologic maw that swallows us up—it runs the intern—the little decisions, **isordil** 5 or 10, sure, those are your decisions, but can I refuse to treat this decrepit demented miserable soul—no way—he's an **ICU hit**—treat now. Sleep later.

At 6:30 a.m. I go to sleep; my demented man **ventilating** away; 45 minutes later I'm up to present my night's work. A good night.

August, 1980

Call me Donald. Some months ago, never mind how long precisely, having nothing to do, and little to interest me on elective, I thought I would pinch hit a little and come back to the ICU. It is a way I have of driving off the spleen and regulating the circulation. Whenever I find myself growing grim about the mouth, whenever it is a damp, drizzly November in my soul, whenever I find myself involuntarily pausing before Room 3, and bringing up the rear in every **code call** I hear, and especially whenever my hypos get such an upper hand of me, that it requires a strong moral principal to prevent me from deliberately coming up to the Bigelow and participating in every disaster. then, I account it high time to get to the unit as soon as I can. This is my substitute for pistol and ball. With a philosophical flourish Cato throws himself upon his sword; I quietly return to the unit. There is nothing surprising in this. If they but knew it, almost all **H.O.s** in their degree sometime or other cherish very nearly the same feeling towards **flogging gomes** as me!

October, 1980

I'm afraid I can't be as enthusiastic as the above contributor. I have just spent my 2nd consecutive night on call **"flogging gomes"**. While there is still the exhilaration of doing things that have dramatic impact (i.e., **shocking** out of **SVT, tubing**, trying a **transvenous pacer**) I can't say that overall I feel good. Last night on call I thought I was going to sleep like a baby - but Noooo! Four **codes** on our team. Not only did the intern not sleep - but the SAR for the house did not sleep. The other SAR on Team A had to get up to push **pronestyl** on the guy who **Vfibbed** X2! (Nurses can't push pronestyl - like you have to have some god-damn MD to push pronestyl!!). Code after code, stable patient after unstable patient - they all went down the tubes. And in the AM when the friendly troops arrive over the horizon - ah!! But then our visit bounces into rounds proclaiming that this is fun! He's sick of "well-baby care." What a pile of shit! Let him stand on his feet with that fucking **lead apron** on for six hours and then have to run back to the unit to handle two more codes!

And last night - things were shaping up pretty well until I get paged to X3321 [the extension for the EW] - a 73-year-old in **pulmonary edema** who doesn't make urine. We've been on our feet literally torturing him with **subclavians**, **cardioversion** out of SVT. And after all our torture he still has a **BP of 40**! And now the sun is up, we're finishing the notes, and the nurses start telling us about the rules "You can't use **Neo w/o an art-line**". "You have to make **the mixes**" - (Why don't they get a Nobel Prize winner in to make the weekend mixes).

March, 1987

Overhead page: "Stat page, **RICU consult**, to the emergency room..."
Dr. S on call today in the ICU: "Oh not now..."
Moments later...
Overhead page: "Stat page, Catholic chaplain, to the emergency room..."
Dr. S, with fists raised: "Saved again!"

A special team of doctors is called by pager and by overhead loudspeakers to every "code blue" in the hospital. The overhead call can also be the MICU resident's first notification of an impending admission: if the patient survives, he or she will be admitted to the MICU.

December, 1986

Dr. M: "This patient is critically ill and has a dismal prognosis—should anything happen we will run a **slow code**."
Dr. J: "So what does that mean—if he **arrests** do we **shock** him?"
Dr. M: "Slowly."

April, 1994

Speaking about a patient in a **neurovegetative state** status post **anoxic brain damage**:
Dr. K: "You mean we still have to **shock** her if she **VF's**?"
Dr. C: "Yes but we don't have to plug in the **defibrillator**."
Dr. K: "Why don't we just hook the defibrillator to a kite with a key and fly the kite out the window?"

A variant of the "slow code."

November, 1998

Rather than holding all of the time-consuming family meetings every day to discuss **status**, we could distribute a generic statement to family members that they could personalize themselves, as demonstrated below:

MICU Madlibs!
We're sorry, but your _____ (name of relative: mother, grandmother, great grandmother) is _____ (fatalistic adverb: horribly, unequivocally, masochistically) ill. In particular his/her (name of body organ: kidney, liver) does not work. Neither does his/her _____ (name of body organ: kidney, liver)... Nor does his/her _____ (name of body organ: kidney, liver). He/she had had a devastating _____ (name of medical event: stroke, MI, bowel

movement). We strongly suggest _____ (verb or verb phrase denoting cessation of efforts: withdrawing, pulling back, stopping the *cheech*) .

June, 1996

Sign Out Rounds.

   ... While discussing a brain-dead patient on whom the plan has changed from **full court press** to **MS0$_4$ drip** because of undulating attending judgement, the team agrees that a place for patients like this, where <u>attendings</u> would cover unit patients, should exist.

   And when deciding on the name of this attending covered unit ... [the response] "how about, "the Fuck U"?

The above entries contain an enormous amount of anger about death and the inability to prevent it, or hasten it.

February, 1990

I nearly always had an awful catch in the throat and three times split at the earliest possible instant to bawl like a child in some bathroom somewhere. You've gotta laugh ...

   And then you just want to be liked and be a part of things and let others know how much you like and love them. And damn it, you just can't seem to make it known. They're all busy and preoccupied. When you stay around to help out they kick you out or they think you're patronizing. And that immense affection just wells up inside with no-where to go... you grow quiet and be your gentle self and they step on you or don't take you seriously. "He's so mild mannered and he always stops to talk to the patient when he's in there- I don't think he's sharp like the others"I heard one nurse say to the other in the hall while I was in with a patient. And sure, there is anger beneath it all that you cannot express and don't wish to acknowledge. Anger over the fact that others don't appreciate you when what you really want is to be loved and valued, anger that people badger you to do things and the more you do the less you're thanked. Anger when someone tells you that you're incredibly slow in presenting patients and then seeing the same person deliver the most conspicuously slow and halting summary of a patient's presenting problems and further care. Anger at the petty digs by others, the minor and major cruelties. But some of the deliberate cruelties practiced here are amazing. I can't bear to be more specific.

There are great moments - you're on top of the world - when you've been congratulated for a fine job, when you've helped a family through a tough time or cleared the confusion, when you see the chance to really help a **H.O.** or nurse or whoever through a bind. It is the unpredictability that is so problematic. We are emotional time bombs, terrible cliché - that it is. Nothing is more vexatious.

Those nights when, maybe at 3AM, you become gradually overtaken by an immense, almost too-great-to-be-contained affection for the people on the ward. Sweet and infinitely mysterious. Incredibly lonely. You feel privileged to be a caretaker - a sort of shepherd guarding the flock. All you want to do is put your arm around the world, to protect.

A few nights back I rode up to the top floor and stole out to the balcony. Sleeping city of concrete, brick, dreams. The world that we serve. The silent sleeping bodies don't know how far up their little lights carry. The city sea. Each night beaching up its quota of ill or unhappy souls on the sands of our **EW.** Who knows what will come. None shall fathom.

It is our inconstancy - inner and outer- that's so problematic. But we've got to remember that we are people, after all and people will sometimes err or fail even in the service of the highest and most binding ideals. We will blow it from time to time - occasionally in truly outstanding style. We may be curt or cranky with our patients: the courses charted by our private lives are not forever smooth or we become affected by the phase of the moon or simply the cantankerousness of an unfed stomach (oh for a Lorna Doone. You'd think it was ambrosia or something - it's all they have here. Except for those grotesque grahams).

And accepting the unacceptable - the times you could strangle your resident, tell the family "If you page me one goddam more time".. or more subtly, it's 4 AM, you've been up all night struggling to keep a man alive. The nurse is at your side as you push **pronestyl** and all you can think of is how much you desire her that instant. The light leaks in with that early morning texture. Life, all of a sudden becomes incredibly cheapened, devalued. You think of the room 3's that didn't make it while you were down in the **Pit,** the chests you pumped on to no avail all the hours spent **"lining"** people, pushing drugs, drawing **gases** all <u>in one night</u>! It's hard to connect to living things and believe that life has meaning. It grows unreal. On seeing the same lady at whose bedside desire suddenly overcame every thought the next day: tremendous respect for a curve of exposed thigh where our hands had trespassed quite rudely for a pulse the night before. Territory known only in loving to a single other. Cure the problem now. Recognize the patient with it later.

The emotional extremes expressed in this single entry are striking – it makes one wonder if the author were post call (and thus, more susceptible to emotional lability) from a particularly harrowing night.

On a more mundane note, saltines, graham crackers, and Lorna Doones are the only foods reliably available on any medical floor.

April, 1983

In a discussion of "celebrity" medicine: "When a president was shot and arrived in the Texas emergency department, everybody was at first in awe. Then they ripped off his clothes and treated him like everybody else."

November, 1985

SAR: "If you find someone **coding** on the street and can't bear to do mouth to mouth, does it do any good to do chest compression?"
Attending: "No! They need oxygen."
SAR: "Then the bottom line is keep on walking."

May, 1985

"I never feel like I really know a patient until I **see his vocal cords**."

February, 1986

A lot of our time is spent flipping in and out of people's rooms - interlopers only - treating the acute disease and often never connecting to the person. The enterprise can grow unreal. Called to see a lifeless form. A **code**. The **EKG** machine unplugged. "Oh shit, another open bed" the intern says. Something died inside me at her remark. We are all too often late comers to pathology's great stage. We arrive sometime near the end of the final act, shortly before the curtain is due to fall, and are asked to alter the play that it might last awhile longer or end more softly. The contrast between the miracles we can sometimes work and our frequent impotence before the fickleness of fate. Humbled and even made strangely peaceful by this.

April, 1980

Richard's law: "If you **buff** the "unbuffable" it's only because he's got another disease that will kill him."

August, 1980

You can't shine shit.

June, 1980

Ladies and gentleman, please take your seats,
The show is about to begin.
Call all the doctors and nurses and **techs**
And notify all next of kin.
It's always the time to perform the next act,
Not ever too early or late.
Their props are in place and the curtain is up.
In the theater **Bigelow 8**.

The theme is familiar. The music begins.
The critical mass will explode
Into the furious blur of a dance
That is danced as the ballet in **code**.

And the colors of code are the pale lucent blue
Of the **gel** that is smeared on the chest.
And the black of the chaplain who hovers about
To make sure the poor bastard is blessed.
And the grain and the brown of the vomit and stool
That are slowly smeared over the bed.
And the blood pumping up in the **ABG tube**
That is always much **blacker than red**.

And the pall that is cast in the room is a hue
That is ghastly cadaverous, cold—
For the purulent breath of the angel of death
Is a terrible sight to behold!

And the sounds of a code are the frightening bell
Shrieking "someone is trying to die."
The clamorous footsteps converge on the site

In their mechanized, practiced reply.
And the call for the lines and the **amps** and the **drips,**
And the sickening thump on the chest,
And the crunching of ribs that are yielding quick,
As the **sternum** is rhythmically pressed.

And a terrible sound that can barely be heard—
It is rasping and harsh and obscene,
As the **agonal** breath of the angel of death
Drools over the fruitless routine.

February, 1980

A sick poem written at a sick time for posterity-

Gomes, gomes, go "avay"
Please, oh please **code** on someone else's day.
On call to pull you from
The clutches of death,
Treating the **lung edema** that
Shortens your breath
Makes me stop and wonder
Just why
Why oh why can't we
Let you comfortably die?
No, of course we won't do that
We'll **flog** you and flog you,
Forever, if it takes that.
Treatment is, of course, the
Order of the day.
What else is medicine for anyway?
We rarely cure and only sometimes
Comfort, but always we treat,

Because otherwise we might
Face Foolish Society's heat.
The people, including ourselves,
Who urge us on, should consider
How they'll feel in twenty years and beyond!

What is it about a code blue that promotes poetry? Perhaps the carefully orchestrated medication protocols; or the rhythm of directions being shouted to the group; or maybe it is a reaction to an event that is anything but poetic.

April, 1991

12:30am ... as I hopped like a bunny?? The candyland trail to gum drop city dropping little gum balls as I go. I'm kind of flaking out. Can you tell, my flathead has orange candy flake glaze the color of crushed gum ball. I keep seeing a crushed nasal septum with oozing blood and I want to make it candy flake, unreal. Everyone around here seems to keep waiting for father time to grim reap them away. Swing low, sweet chariot, four angels in black face doing a # over several beds tonight. Hold on ZAAAPPPPP flop.

Lets cut out that kind of stuff, This is no half court game, it's a **full court press** you gotta believe in 1% **prognosis**.

Bring, Bring, Bring. Hello this is Mortimer Snerd of the Forked Tongue Tasting Society and I wondered if you could tell me, possibly let me know if you would be interested in one of our true blue for you to clues to the screws that dues and don'ts of baby my time I guess I'll never be here again. It's kind of nice at this point.

June, 1993

Last Night in the You Nit

46

I just reread all my old notes in the book. They all seemed to reflect some sadness, fear and wild excitability. That was internship. Internship and the unit, that first summer was also quite lonely. Everything was very unfamiliar. Starting to get sloppy again. Scent - o- mint pop one you too can freshen your breath doublemint commercial. Can you see their lips smacking. Looking out the window over Boston lights and the **Bulfinch** view I just I just can't believe it is all over. This is really the last night. I can hear the hum of the vacuums in the EW coffee room at 3:00 a.m. I can see that first night when a nurse started an **IV** for me at 3:00 a.m. I can feel the fear in the pit of my stomach when another resident and I **coded** this poor sucker with **V-tach** in the elevator. On the way up from the **pit**. I can't forget when one nurse cried like a baby when this sensitive psychoanalyst died. I can't forget another resident, **intubating** an 80-year-old man with end stage prostatic cancer and horrible bone pain. Zapppp Pow Kabow. Now be careful, you are getting too concrete. How can one be sure that you truly remember what happens!

You were a **toxic 'tern**, your mind must have been soft like an egg half soft and half hard boiled, ready to hatch. Fly away, fly away my little chickadee. I can see W.C. Fields on the beach, it's an endless summer Brian Wilson and the boys doing surfer girl on the beach! Like let's hop in our Woodies till Daddy takes the **TB** away. You say that your wings are gone that Jan and Dean wiped out at Dead Man's curve. Whooh are you going to cop out about that old class argument. I mean AIDS doesn't affect nice boys and girls. Thank god that Johnny's college extension kept him off the Ho Chi Minh trail.

Too late for this idealistic mumbling. Or perhaps you don't think I really give a shit. Yes I do. More than ever I feel that I am a physician and still care. That is what makes me happy and know that it is finally time to leave. Training time is over. Goodbye, Yawl.

A lucid, thoughtful, self-reflective entry, on his final night in the MICU, from the author of other, somewhat incomprehensible stream-of-consciousness entries.

September, 1993

The JAR, on entering an elderly patient's room and tidying him up -amid his lines and tubes – hears a yelp: "Are you unplugging me?"

June, 1981

I guess the heart gets used to beating and is slow to stop.

CHAPTER THREE:

Humor

Few things cut through tension as quickly as humor. I remember watching a staff neurologist examine a critically ill, 70-year-old man with a recent stroke; the patient was unresponsive to questions and lacked any spontaneous movement. The neurologist's task was to determine the patient's prognosis for a meaningful life. During the examination the patient's cardiac monitor alarm sounded emitting a loud musical tone. Without missing a beat the neurologist looked up from testing the man's reflexes, and said, "Does that mean I win the car?" Laughter erupted from other doctors and nurses in attendance. Seconds later, cardiopulmonary resuscitation (CPR) was initiated. The concern for a man on the brink of life, juxtaposed with a sudden alarm that sounded like a tune played on a TV game show, was striking. The brief bout of levity reduced the somber atmosphere that surrounded the patient. Though the neurologist's humorous remark was unplanned, as is often the case with humor, it had a temporary salutary effect.

Most people recognize humor when they see it; but they neither understand why something is funny nor realize its benefits. Humor is not unidimensional; it comes in myriad shapes and styles. Variably defined as a comic quality causing amusement, humor often involves the recognition and expression of incongruities present in situations or characters.

Crude and insensitive humor is often used to illustrate fundamental absurdities in human nature or conduct. Frequently driven by anger or danger, it may convey thinly-veiled threats or sexual desires. Bathroom humor, which employs references to human excrement and to sexual organs, is one such example. Wit is a more intellectual type of humor, characterized by cleverness, wordplay, and and sharp observations or remarks.

Humor is context dependent: its effectiveness is determined by who is around when the humor is displayed. For example, if a 10-year-old places two straws in his nostrils while in conversation with his friends, this may be very funny. But if a physician were to do it while in the room of a critically-ill person surrounded by family, it probably would not be met with smiles. Few physicians can pull off outrageous humor or slapstick comedy and get away with it. Patch Adams could, but most MICU doctors have neither the creativity nor the sense of timing of Dr. Adams.

While reading ostensibly humorous diary entries in this book, it is important to remember that what is funny to one person or group may not be funny to another. It may help to put yourself into the MICU residents' shoes. Imagine that you've been awake for 24-36 hours, you haven't had a day off in 3 weeks, you've had very little time outside of the hospital for socializing with friends or family, and you find yourself having to make life and death decisions on a daily basis. Wouldn't you want a break? Rather than say to an ICU physician ", How can you joke while my father is dying?" Think, "How can you not invoke humor?" The physician's behavior belies the fact that he is sensitive to the juxtaposition of critical illness and absurdity.

Humor can also be used as a vehicle for teaching. When I try to explain to staff the phenomenology of delirium, or acute brain failure (often manifested by episodic inattention, agitation, confusion, memory problems, and hallucinations), I can't help but think of this story of two truck drivers: "One trucker didn't think his blinkers were working so he stopped the truck and asked the other trucker to get out and check them. When he got out of the truck and inspected the blinkers, he said, 'They're working, they're not working, they're working, they're not working...'" Obviously, that's what blinkers do when they are functional. With delirium, the patient will be clear and thoughtful one moment, and then episodically agitated and confused. It is the very pattern of episodic agitation and confusion that leads one to the diagnosis of delirium and to a search for potential etiologies; then specific treatment can be initiated as rapidly as possible.

Most physicians and other people-- patients-- relish a physician with a sense of humor. Having a sense of humor does not prevent a physician from taking a situation seriously. In fact, it is the presence of humor that may enable him or her to cope. In the MICU humor bonds staff. Sleep, food, and shared laughter are powerful medicines and great pacifiers. Displays of humor insulate staff from the misery around them and allow them to tolerate tragic circumstances. A MICU team that lacks a sense of humor often feels tortured by the endless rounding and by the burden of caring for the sick. Staff yearn for the equivalent of the class clown, and for the opportunity to laugh instead of cry. Far from interfering with care, levity allows doctors to recognize a tragic situation and focus on treating their patients. While a certain amount of emotional intensity may heighten attention and promote focus, when the emotional load becomes too great, the resulting anxiety or dread may become debilitating. At that point, a physicians needs the relief of comedy, as an escape valve, to function as a healer again.

Humor breaks the tension of emotionally draining ICU work, and the MICU culture demands it. However, to outsiders, the gallows humor (a type of humor that makes fun of a very serious or terrifying situation) that is displayed may seem inappropriate, sophomoric, and ill timed. It probably is.

Our hope is to share with you the varieties of humor employed in the MICU. Our intent is not to condone insensitivity, but to place humor in the MICU in perspective. Humor can facilitate coping, but it comes with a price.

Theodore A. Stern, M.D.

October, 1994

On call, Dr. W, as prepared as always, opens his overnight bag. Something buzzes and vibrates the whole table. Blushing, he stuffs the object into his pocket. "It's a razor really," the heavily-bearded intern states.

January, 1988

Trying to assess the Thomas' ages, the ICU team notes the following:
JAR: "The Thomas' have been married for 13 years."
Intern: "13 years!!! They got married when I was 14 years old. I wonder what I was doing when I was 14..."
JAR: "I know what you were doing. That's why your eyesight isn't so good."

August, 1998

The JAR, while comforting a patient during an **A-line flog**, turned around and set the TV on the soft porn channel--she said softly. . . "Oh my!"

December 23, 1992

Dr. D--while Santa occupied a bed in the MICU (**intubated** and paralyzed): "Actually, I slept with Santa last night."
Intern: "Does Santa need a Psychiatry Consult after last night?"
Dr. E: "No, but he needs a rape test."

An MGH tradition: A life-sized Santa Claus doll is "admitted" in mid-December, having suffered a holiday-related calamity (e.g., mad reindeer disease, antler impalement), and always leaving the hospital December 24, against medical advice.

February, 1986

Drs. V and H, both with a cold, discussing if they should look at their **sputum gram stains**: "I'll look at yours if you'll look at mine."

September, 1996

Intern: "You know, I once gave a guy a penile spasm."
SAR: "I don't want to hear about your social life."

November, 1992

Team: "Risk factors for **aortic dissection**?"
JAR: "Syphilis."
Team: "How could you have known that?"
JAR: "Well, my social life was better before internship!"

October, 1991

Sign-out rounds:
Dr. G: "C'mon let's hurry up."
JAR: "Why, do you have a life outside the hospital? What's the rush?"
Dr. G: "Sometimes..."
Intern: "That's because G is married!"
Dr. R: "I wish I could have seen you dance in junior high school..."

March, 1989

JAR: "You guys are so out of it; you don't know what 'funky col' medina' is!"
Intern: "What is it?"
JAR: "I can't believe you don't know—it was the number one song in the country!"

Intern: "That's because we don't date high school girls."

February 14, 1997

Dr. S, reading from the little Valentine's Day candies:
"One kiss--" Ooh, I really scored!"
Dr. O: "S, one kiss is not really scoring."
Dr. S: "Oh, I should have dated you in high school."

When push comes to shove, particularly when sleep deprivation and patient acuity increases, humor related to the themes of sex and violence abound.

January, 1999

A discussion took place regarding the possible complications of giving **Epinephrine**.
SAR: "Well, you can **necrose** peripheral parts of the body, like the nose, the penis, or the fingers."
JAR: "I know which of those I would choose last. Does size matter in that situation?"
SAR: "Of course it does-- if you want to have something left. . . "

May, 1987

After the team joked about Dr. Y's **post-partum** figure, she promised to show off her body by wearing a string bikini the next morning. "But," she added, "I'll bring a bottle of **Compazine** to pass out to the team!"

December 1991

On morning rounds, the JAR on the road to matrimony, plans for a future: "Let's see, if I get pregnant right now, I wouldn't have the baby until August."
SAR: "It would also make rounds a little uncomfortable for the rest of us."
(The JAR agrees to perform "the act" outside of the **Death Star**).

April, 1987

The JAR, commenting on the **urologists**: "They take care of a very small part of medicine."
SAR: "Speak for yourself!"

October, 1990

On sign-out rounds the nurse approached the conference room.
Nurse: "Mr. E has that thing in his...uh...penis and...uh...well, I can't get the...uh...foreskin back."
Dr. R: "Well...Dr. U (A **urologist**) is used to seeing these problems, and I'm sure he can take care of it."
JAR (to Dr. R): "Yes, Dr. R wouldn't know about 'these problems' because he's Jewish!!
Dr. R: "Okay...so we'll get a stat *moyle* consult."

May, 1993

SAR (to a cardiologist): "You know Mr. Z, he's your private patient."
Cardiologist: "I know his **groin**, not his face!"

August, 1983

The JAR, presenting a case of a young overdose patient on visit rounds: "On physical exam, he was a large tanned muscular strapping..."
Dr. A: "And those were only a few of the adjectives in the chart...."
SAR: "Why did it take you and the intern so long to work him up?"
JAR: (flushed, embarrassed) "Thank God my husband isn't here."
Dr. A: "Do you have a big strapping husband?"
JAR: "No but I have a big strapping dog."
Attending: "He apparently isn't the kind of guy you'd bring home to dinner."
SAR: "At least not without calling first."
JAR: "Yeah, so my Mom could get a shotgun."
Intern: "Well, I don't know. At this point my Mom might not object so strongly...."
JAR: "Well, when I went to see him he had been stripped and was lying in four-point restraints with his legs over the sides of the stretcher—at least I covered him with a sheet instead of uncovering him!"
Intern: "I was looking for his **femoral artery**!!"
Chorus: "That's what they all say!"

Cardiac catheterizations are performed to diagnose and treat coronary artery disease. These procedures involve placement of catheters into the femoral artery and/or vein, located in the groin. The catheter is then threaded up the vessels that coarse through the abdomen and chest, leading back to the heart. Once in the heart, a dye is injected to visualize the coronary vessels and the function of the heart muscle itself, using a special x-ray machine. Rare complications of this procedure include bleeding at the site of catheter insertion (i.e., in the groin). To monitor the patient for these complications, either the resident or the cardiologist checks a patient's groin frequently.

March, 1998

An MGH psychologist was in the ICU following her successful **PTCA**. She was in good spirits and thought she'd tell the team a joke. She said: "An elderly couple both in their 80s had just gotten married. On their honeymoon night they each gradually undressed taking off one article of clothing at a time. The woman was down to her panties and about to take them off and climb into bed when she told her new husband, 'I have to warn you, I have acute angina,' to which her husband replied, 'I sure hope so 'cause the rest of you isn't so nice!'"

The team laughed, and the JAR who was on call and waiting to examine her said, "Okay ma'am I have to look at your groin now."

June, 1991

A series of William Kennedy Smith jokes ensues. "What's the sign outside the Palm Springs Kennedy house say?" "Trespassers will be violated." Haha.
Then: "He said, don't tell or I'll have my uncle drive you home."
Intern: "Oh yeah, I get it, Chattanooga!"
The JAR, unable to contain himself: "That's Chappaquidick, you numbnut!"

September, 1992

Attending: "Orthopaedics has a mnemonic for counting your ribs: "1, 2, 3, 4 . . ."
And…
"The hardest two years of an orthopedist's life is 1st grade."

June, 1984

"The only difference between your hands and a surgeon's hands is that yours are connected to a brain."

Patients are not the only targets of doctors' frustrations and humor. Barbed attacks are also directed at colleagues.

January, 1991

The SAR, concerned about a patient's failure to defecate over the past 4-5 days: "He needs to stool, stool, stool!"
The attending rhetorically states: "Don't be a stool pigeon!"

May, 1993

Attending: "Alcoholic **CNS** effects?"
Intern: "Short-term . . . you get drunk!"
Attending: "He's got to stick to what he knows!"

July, 1988

Attending: "I can't understand it! A trained chimp could get down that **bronchus**."
SAR: "I think even the JAR could get down it."
Attending: "I said trained."

January, 1989

The attending, commenting on moving a patient from the **vent** to measure the **wedge**: "Who is the cretin who did that—that person needs to have his **TSH** checked."

Cretinism is a condition of low iodine intake which causes an under-active thyroid (hypothyroidism), dwarfism, and mental retardation. In fact, the word cretin derives from the Franco-Provencal word crestin, or Christian, as sufferers of this condition were considered so profoundly retarded as to be incapable of sin.

April, 1991

It's hard to soar like an eagle when you fly with turkeys.

November, 1991

"Opinions are like assholes. Everyone has one and everyone else's stinks."

May, 1980

Question: What is the difference between an intern and a pile of shit?
Answer: People will go out of their way not to step on the pile of shit.

May, 1984

"The national flower in this ICU is the hedge."

August, 1992

The attending, angry with himself for forgetting the details of a *New England Journal of Medicine* reference:
Attending: "I'm suffering from the CRS syndrome."
Team: "What's CRS syndrome?"
Attending: "Can't remember shit syndrome."

As in many professions, TLAs, or "Three-letter Acronyms," are used to distance members of the profession from those outside of the profession. The professionals often view them as time-savers, when is reality they may be more important as forms of fraternal bonding.

June, 1984

SAR: "What's the difference between **acute** and **chronic aortic insufficiency**?"
Intern: "One's acute and one's chronic! "

November, 1993

On Rounds, SAR: "A, trade with E so I can see the **flow sheets**."
Dr. A: "What? You don't like being next to me?"
SAR: "Not when you smell that way."
Dr. A: "But I change my underpants once a week!"
SAR: "Changing them front to back doesn't count as changing them."

February, 1993

After hearing a patient presentation:
Attending: "Okay. Nice job. Let's go to the bedside."
Intern: "What's at the bedside?"
JAR: "Oh yeah. The patient."

October, 1981

Team-**visit** interaction at its best:
Visit: "He's had **bronchitis** and **hemoptysis** three times in the past, so now he has bronchitis and hemoptysis and you want to rule out **P.E.** It looks like a duck, quacks like a duck, smells like a duck, so what is it? A duck!"

Team: "**Rule out** chicken!"

When a patient comes to the hospital with a complaint, it is the doctor's job to consider all of the potential causes of the complaint, and then "rule-out" the more unlikely ones, in coming to a final diagnosis. For example, causes of a patient's complaint of chest pain could include a heart attack, a pneumonia, indigestion, or an anvil having fallen on the patient's chest. Questions must be asked to refine the diagnostic possibilities, and laboratory tests considered. If the patient with chest pain has not experienced cough, fever, or a recent ingestion of a spicy meal, then pneumonia and indigestion probably can be "ruled-out." If there is no evidence of recent trauma, then the patient's chest pain is unlikely to be the result of an anvil-induced accident. This does not mean that the cause of the chest pain is definitely a heart attack, but it makes it a more likely possibility.

August, 1992

Dr. M (describing a patient with **change in mental status**): "she would intermittently break into spontaneous laughter in the absence of stimuli. . . "
SAR: "If you call Dr. M's jokes absence of stimuli. . . ."

August, 1983

The JAR, about a patient's **mental status** at 1 a.m.: "He was difficult to arouse but no more so than my wife is at 1 a.m."

February, 1992

On morning rounds, when word was made of the fact that the SAR was going into Cardiology, the Attending said: "A mind is a terrible thing to waste."

SAR: "Yes, but a dollar is a wonderful thing to spend."

March, 1981

"**Neurologists** don't treat disease—they admire it."

May, 1992

"I hate antibiotics. They destroy the natural course of all great diseases."

November, 1998

JAR: "Ms. R is now on **meripenim, Liposomal Ampho, Vancomycin**, and **Chloramphenicol**."
SAR: "Why don't we just lose the antibiotics and **Autoclave** him?"

July 1996

Comment by the JAR, in referring to the **poly-antimicrobial** regimen of a patient who had an infection with no source: "Well, I guess we've got everything covered, except maybe maggots!"

When faced with a critically-ill patient whose clinical presentation suggests infection, most physicians will initiate treatment with one or more antibiotics. The risk of waiting for the correct identification of the infectious source before antibiotics are begun outweighs the risk of giving a potentially unnecessary medicine.

December, 1996

Discussing a diabetic patient who was normally admitted with her seeing-eye dog, but who now is a denizen of the MICU.

Intern: "I don't think she could have glass eyes because she's described as 'legally blind.' Those are the people who you say, 'You really shouldn't drive' to, not the ones with **bilateral** prosthetic eyes. . . "
SAR: "Have you ever driven in Boston?"

July, 1984

While discussing ways to maximize the likelihood of **extubation** while weaning a 450-pound patient, the JAR suggested an orthopedic consult to institute breast traction. "Nothing like getting a load off your chest!"

The residents here are using humor to solidify their knowledge of pulmonary mechanics and ventilator management. A person who is obese has a harder time breathing on a ventilator because the weight of his own chest presses down on the lungs, making them harder to inflate.

January, 1996

On the morning of the day that a family decision was to be made on Mr. E's status, an unfortunate gentleman whom we **cheeched** for weeks, we hear that the son (the spokesman) is at an outside hospital, with possible appendicitis.

The JAR, exasperated on hearing this, comments: "Pray for **Mittelschmertz**!"

The resident hopes for the absurd, as men cannot get Mittelschmertz, an intermenstrual pain that would not keep a woman in the hospital.

June, 1985

The SAR, describing her research which involves studying the **endocrine** cycle of cows.

SAR: "You strap on a long glove and examine the ovaries to tell where they are in the cycle."
JAR: "Sounds like a big deal. Can't you just ask them to keep records?"

December, 1996

Concerning possible alternates to **conducting gel** (during codes where they never can find "the goo"), the JAR noted, "So, the old wives' tale about using butter with the **paddles** is untrue?"

Aptil, 1991

The JAR, responding to the visiting chief resident's question, "So what kind of monitoring system do you have here on **White 8**?"
JAR: "We choose the patient's roommates carefully."

August, 1998

The JAR, referring to a patient: "He's having a ton of blood from his butt, he's just having a huge amount of blood from his butt."

Dr. B, usually a rather quiet intern, leans over her shoulder and adds, as if for clarification: "From his butt hole."

February, 1992

Intern: "She was up in the chair today, rockin' on the bedpan. She looks like a rose!"
JAR: "I saw her, she does not look like a rose. And she definitely didn't smell like one."

June, 1982

Intern: "She was found in the supermarket, frothing at the mouth."

SAR: "This was unusual for her?"

March, 1994

In reference to the hooker who reportedly has a seizure disorder—
Nurse: What if she seizes while turning a trick?
Intern: Some guy will go away mighty impressed with himself!

January, 1983

Dr. U, on a patient who survived a **VF arrest** and had post-arrest **myoclonus** and seizures: "Maybe we should just put him in front of K Mart and let the kids put coins in his eyes and ride the rides."

In the MICU, outrageous and sick humor, while insensitive and not likely to be considered socially acceptable, can be funny. To whom it is funny depends on which side of the street, or what side of the patient's bed, you are on. As described in the essay beginning this chapter, gallows' humor serves many functions.

November, 1981

Regarding a 20-year-old woman with the habit of coming in with **DKA** after running out of money for food:
Dr. L: "What's the matter with her boyfriend, why doesn't he feed her?.. She must be a really cheap date."

June, 1982

"The patient had a **blood sugar of 29...differential diagnosis** included Von Bulow's syndrome."

Sunny Von Bulow was an affluent Newport socialite who was found comatose in association with an extremely low blood sugar level that was allegedly caused by insulin injections.

February, 1991

On a.m. work rounds: On a patient who has been a diagnostic puzzle:
Attending: "What' the patient's travel history recently?"
JAR: "To radiology and back!"

Unusual infectious diseases can be caused by exposure to bacteria, viruses, and parasites in exotic lands. As a result, physicians often inquire about travel histories.

April, 1987

With a **PO$_2$** in the teens and a **PCO$_2$** in the hundreds, she's one of the reasons the rest of us can breathe....she actually puts O$_2$ back in the environment. She has **xylem and phloem** in her veins.

August, 1988

The intern, presenting a new patient: "It just seems that she is in a bad social situation."
Attending: "Well, it's hard to enjoy a party when you're **intubated**."

November, 1983

The SAR, on a family's objections to "pulling the plug" on an 80-year-old **gome**: "We won't pull the plug—we'll just pull the tube and leave the machine going."

An interesting end-run solution to a thorny problem.

April, 1990

On morning rounds, nurse frustrated over hard of hearing, demented patient: "I just told him not to tug at his **Foley**, but he's still holding on to it, asking me, "When can I let go of the tube?"
Attending: "More than three shakes is a sin."

September, 1986

The SAR, in reference to a patient going home with a **suprapubic tube** in place: "Oh boy—better not get that one caught in the car door."

June, 1989

When discussing Mr. C:
Intern: "He was incontinent. He has trouble with the **Texas catheter**."
JAR: "Is it too big for him?"
Intern: "Yeah—he needs a Rhode Island catheter."

June, 1984

Dr. B, referring to a somewhat agitated and demented patient who was pulling on his **Foley**: "He's definitely better; he's pulling on the right organ."

May, 1983

"For his protection we have to tighten this **restraint order**, because either he will pull his **Foley** out or he will pull his penis off."

October, 1986

In visit rounds discussing a patient who pulled out his **Foley** with the **balloon up**:

Attending: "You never know your limits until you're pushed."
JAR: "....or pulled..."

March, 1989

With regards to a patient with a penile prosthesis, the SAR remarks, "He's in permanent **wedge**."

The medical equivalent of bathroom humor is always good for a laugh. Foley catheters are rubber tubes inserted through the urethra and into the bladder, to drain urine. To anchor them in the bladder, a balloon at the catheter tip is inflated once the catheter has been inserted.

Penile prostheses come in different forms. One type is inflatable; this action is similar to that of pulmonary artery catheters, intended to measure heart function.

September, 1993

JAR (sarcastically), on a **Road Warrior**: "He was admitted to the floor and immediately **lost to follow-up**.

October, 1985

In attempting to transfer a marine veteran to a VA hospital:
JAR: "They won't accept him until they're sure he's a vet."
SAR: "Let's send him over in a uniform."

January, 1983

Theoretically speaking, she's better off than most 93-year-old women. But then again most 93-year-old women are dead.

July, 1997

The SAR to Mr. V, who had a **post-cath**. complication of **pericarditis**:
"Does it hurt when you breathe?"
"Yes."
"Then, don't do that."

December, 1996

Discussing an unfortunate patient who suffered severe burn to her chest wall while putting a log in her fireplace, the Attending suggests we obtain a recreation consult.

October, 1991

After massive **hematemesis**, profuse **melena**, and several **syncopal** episodes, Mr. C states that he "crawled to the **T** and went home," prompting the JAR to observe:
"You can usually get a seat on the T if you pass melena."

For some people, the desire to be in the comfort of their own homes is paramount. Notice also how the resident distances himself from the severity of the situation by focusing on a minor aspect of the story.

March, 1987

Discussing Mr. R, 400-pound patient with **respiratory arrest**, lower extremity **cellulitis**, the SAR inquires about what grew out of his cellulitis **aspirate**. The Intern was quick to provide the essential information: "Twinkies."

Few things generate anger in young physicians as much as self-inflicted illness.

August, 1992

A 59-year-old woman with alcoholic **cirrhosis**, cervical cancer, ovarian cancer, had an ammonia level of 470.
The SAR comments: "Wow, she qualifies as an industrial cleaner."

May, 1994

After undergoing the all-out **neuro/endocrine cheech**, we are told to check Mr. L's aluminum level. The SAR queries: "If it comes back high does that mean we can recycle him?"

April, 1997

With the amount of yeast in Mr. O's urine, that's not urine he's making, it's beer!"

April, 1991

The Attending, on Mrs. E's yeast **UTI**: "We could probably sell her urine to a bread company."

September, 1998

Intern: "Jeez, this new admission has a huge psychiatric history."
SAR: "So, I guess his **VT** was just a cry for help."

June 26, 1996

Best first day quote by the JAR (said of unresponsive patient): L's **mental status** is much better, but I still wouldn't want her as my Quiz Bowl partner!"

January, 1984

Patient to the SAR: "We'd like to have our father cremated when he dies."
The SAR's reply: "If his fever keeps up the way it's been, he may do it himself."

July, 1994

The JAR regarding Mrs. B, a confused elderly woman, who last night thought she was in a recreation room in the pool/sauna and playing pool. "She was having more fun in that room than I have most of my vacations."

House officers who work extended hours often bemoan the fact that they've lost the ability to enjoy an active social life.

February, 1998

On a pneumonia patient:
"Why isn't he extubated yet?"
"Dermatology has to come by to do the little skin prick to see if he has a reaction to the mold he was cleaning."
"Didn't they come by yet?"
"No, it's that short guy."
"So, we're just waiting around for that little prick. . ."

August, 1994

Dr. Y, regarding a patient who had an acute **IMI** while watching the Red Sox lose again: "Jeez,??? you'd think he would have **tachyphylaxed** to that by now."

December, 1981

The Intern, coming into the ICU team to patient: "Hi—I'm the new doctor on the team."
Patient to the Intern: "Well you'll get used to it pretty soon."

March, 1996

The SAR was doing community work last night in East Boston. He asked his team of guardians to list alternatives to "doing drugs." I quote verbatum:

Go to the movies
Play Play Station.
Play ball
Pool
Getting arrested
Safe sex
Ping-Pong
Phone sex
Swimming
Skinny-dipping
Someone whip you
You whip someone's ass.

What the Hell am I doing here?

October, 1984

"Mass General is like Alice in Wonderland." As the Cheshire cat said to Alice, "You can't be normal, you're here and we are all crazy here!"

May, 1998

The SAR, responding to a patient's **pH of 7.21**:
"Don't worry, he lives down there in acid land."
JAR: "Aren't those the lyrics you wrote for Springstein, "living down there in acidland"?

August, 1997

"Did you use a **Walrus** to **cannulate** the femoral vein? "
"I used an eggman."

January, 1984

The Attending, after an intricate discussion on the biochemical nuances of **DKA**: "Besides, the whole point of the body is to supply enough glucose to the brain...so we can fantasize."

August, 1993

SAR: "How was your night ?"
Intern: "Great, I slept through the night!"
JAR: "What?! The nurses woke me up every 15 minutes."
Intern: "Yeah, I've got a trick . . . I sleep naked.!"
(And the nurses are too scared to enter the room).

April, 1990

The Attending, on dealing with Mrs. E's husband (former surgeon): "So, I get this phone call from Dr. E asking, "Are you seeing my wife?"

May, 1996

The Pulmonary Fellow assesses comatose patients in **neurovegetative states** withdrawal to pain, with an easily reproducible test--the titty twister--that would raise the dead from the grave.

In reviewing Levy's criteria (*JAMA*, 1995), we found that no response to titty twister was only predictive of no recovery from vegetative state in conjunction with the **gold standard**: No spontaneous eye movement to the super-wedgie.

Despite the serious nature of profound neurologic dysfunction, physicians often respond with "humor." Several pain-inducing diagnostic maneuvers have been considered to establish the alertness of the unresponsive patient. Some as yet unaccepted and sadistic interventions have been contemplated, but are rarely, if ever, invoked.

February, 1985

On rounds, the Attending was explaining to the team the concept of Hobson's Choice. "Hobson was a stable owner, and all the gentry came to his stable to ride...and when it came to which horse they got, it would be 'Hobson's Choice'—the next available horse. So you see Hobson's Choice is like having a choice when you don't really have a choice at all."

Pause.

Then I asked, "Is that like soup of the day?"

July, 1984

The SAR, on an 81-year-old woman who had a **V-tach arrest** in a courtroom: "Some people will use any excuse to get out of jury duty."

November, 1986

I have never hit a patient, except in anger.

February, 1988

The Intern to Mrs. W: "And how are you feeling today?"
Mrs. W: "With my hands, of course."
The SAR says to the team: "That settles it. Put the **tube** back in!"

May, 1991

The team discussed whether to move one of two patients who intensely dislike each other from their double room.
SAR: "Let's move Mrs. S. She feels claustrophobic."
Intern: "Why don't we just move Ms. C. Then the room will be less crowded."
SAR: "Why not just shoot one of them."
Intern: "Great idea. Isn't that the off-tern's job?"

When taken out of context, outrageous suggestions seem harsher than they were intended to be. Absurd solutions to difficult problems alleviate tension, but are not implemented.

March, 1993

Speaking of Mr. B (420 lbs.) "If this guy were a cow, he'd make for great ribs."

Dehumanizing, isn't it?

May, 1983

"Whenever there is an orifice, there's a will. And whenever there's a will, there's a way."

And whenever there's a will, there's relatives.

June, 1981

Presenting a case that was discharged 1 day before.
JAR: "You'll want to hear about this case for legal reasons...you may get called 9 months from now."
Attending: "What...did you make her pregnant?"

July, 1992

The Attending, on Mrs. R's on-again, off-again recurrence of nausea and vomiting: "She's not yorking, she's New Yorking."

February, 1986

On a patient, 49-year-old man with extensive **anterolateral MI**, someone noted: "The cat's already out of the barn."
Later, Dr. N on such expressions: "That's a fish of a different color. Or maybe another kettle of horses."

Dumb, nonsensical humor may reflect exhaustion, mental dullness, insensitivity, or stupidity.

December 25, 1987

Code bells ring, are you listening?
In the rooms, vents are hissing.

It's a beautiful sight,
We are happy tonight.
On call in the MICU wonderland.

October, 1991

The JAR to Mr. K (an 84-year-old man admitted at 6:30 a.m., **intubated** post-**acute respiratory failure** and agitated, having **anxiolytic** pushed): "Remember, sir, Valium is **amnestic**."

June, 1982

Regarding a patient with diffuse **fibrotic lung** changes, pneumonia and **ARDS:**
Attending: "The chest x-ray does not show an **infiltrate**, even today, but you could hide a house in those lungs."
JAR: "Yeah, but I wouldn't want to take a mortgage out on it."

May, 1996

A patient is flown from Frankfurt to London with a **basilar infarct** now **vent-dependent** and unresponsive. He is flown from London to MGH now **hypotensive** and on **pressors**. Plan: To fly him home to Arkansas.
SAR: "Well he's as ready as he'll ever be. We've called for an air ambulance to come get him."
Intern: "Gee will there be a movie on the flight?"
SAR: "Yeah. I hear it's 'Coma'."

May, 1984

Speaking about Mr. L, a psychotic, demented, **depruned** 81-year-old man with **Parkinson's**.

JAR: "I think he will be ready to **fly** by Monday."
SAR (in quick reply): "Yes, but will he have a place to land?"

October, 1994

JAR: "Let's run Mr. M's issues. . . Oh, wait, we have a late-breaking **gas**."
SAR: "Oh, I have that problem sometimes too."

June, 1997

Everybody **spikes** here. It's like a fucking volleyball game.

February, 1982

On morning rounds, discussing a patient with **CLL**, and **sepsis**.
JAR: "I'm going to call social service today. I understand that the patient doesn't have a home; he lives in a camper with his wife."
SAR: "Where did you learn this?"
JAR: "From his son. He says he thinks his father is very depressed."
SAR: "Does that mean he's not a happy camper?"

March, 1996

Intern: "We should check bedside **pulmonary function tests** in Mr. N, even though they're going to suck."
JAR: "Don't you mean blow?"

February, 1986

The Intern after an abusive night, presenting a patient on rounds: "The patient was a 60-year-old woman with an **endotrachial tube** alert and oriented."

"I hope the **ET tube** wasn't moving all its extremities as well."

The last thing the post-call intern wishes to hear after 30 hours without sleep is a correction of his grammar..

October, 1982

As Shakespeare said when examining his first patient with **pericarditis**: "Ah....there's the **rub**."

November, 1987

The SAR and Intern on an ICU patient with possible **cavitations** on chest x-ray and possible right-sided **endocarditis**.
SAR: "What do you do when you see **vegetations**?"
Intern: "Make salad."

The use of word play and the double-meaning of selected words is intended to minimize the severity of a patient's critical cardiac illness.

November, 1987

The Intern, presenting on a homeless patient with alcohol abuse.
"The EW write up read, 'smelly Reeboks.'"
SAR: "Hmm...toxic sock syndrome."

April, 1985

Said of the German lady who **aspirated** a sausage and went home the next day: "Boy, she was a fast '**weiner**'."

March, 1990

Commenting on a patient just status-post **AKA**, The JAR said, "Looks like she's one leg up on us today!"

Physicians use humor, because at times it is easier to laugh than to cry.

February, 1994

The Attending, commenting on a patient recovering from a profound **methanol** overdose, with a **pH of 6.79** and **bicarb of 1**:
JAR: "He said he had run out of vodka, and thought that a few shots of aftershave wouldn't hurt."
Attending: "Would you say he's had a close shave?"

June, 1981

"It's better to be pissed off than pissed on."

This statement summarizes much of the philosophy conveyed by the above entries.

CHAPTER FOUR

On Life and Death

Most physicians, whether they are practitioners of internal medicine or specialize in oncology, cardiology, or a branch of surgery, confront death. However, in any medical practice, the further away one gets from caring for hospitalized patients, the less often one faces death and the dying. In the MICU every patient is in critical condition, and death is a near daily occurrence.

At the MGH, the MICU team cares for 18 patients at a time; each patient's life is in jeopardy. In part because of this clinical load, physicians rarely act like, or take the time to act like, Marcus Welby (who seemed to have only one patient each week). By contrast with Dr. Welby, our MICU physicians may at first blush appear cold, uncaring, and insensitive--and at times they are. They are also, by and large, younger, less likely to have experienced loss in their lifetime, and more stressed by long work hours, by endless demands, and by chronic sleep deprivation. However, they are not Cub Scouts. The MICU physicians are among the most experienced in applying the technologies and techniques necessary to care for the critically ill and are better prepared for this than most physicians who provide primarily outpatient care. Unfortunately, it is difficult to remain sensitive in the face of the conditions under which they toil, and it is problematic to receive rigorous and empathic training while on the frontlines. Fortunately, they work alongside nurses in the MICU. Nurses are immersed in the daily bedside care of critically ill patients and have extended contacts with family and friends. Little escapes the eyes of an experienced MICU nurse who spends 8-12 hours a day with his or her patient. They see the telling exchanges between visitors and the patient, and deal with issues of comfort, and communication. Such stresses, however, also put them at risk for burnout. As an advocate for the patient, some nurses push physicians to be less ambiguous and to make difficult life and death decisions. No one wants to see someone they have cared for suffer. Emotions run high when the specter of death looms large. Hopelessness, hostility, anxiety, fear, depression, and guilt are common, as is denial, which may be preferred to other emotional states. This gamut of emotions can occur not only in patients, their families, and friends, but also in the doctors and nurses who care for them, if they allow these feelings to rise to the surface. Some patients, their families, and friends, are intolerant of the inevitable; they neither face nor accept the reality of dying. Their irritability and isolation may complicate care and jeopardize treatment.

Some people entering the MICU bring with them conflicts over abandonment. The threat of separation brought on by death heightens these conflicts and makes interpersonal interactions difficult in a variety of ways. Distortions often develop when bad news is provided; accusations and exhibitions of selfishness may arise.

Dying is not always sudden; typically, it is neither neat nor clean. Lines and tubes are uncomfortable fixtures in the MICU patient's world. Patients with end-stage conditions must endure complications of the dying process: depression, delirium, pain, weakness, nausea, vomiting, shortness of breath, a lack of privacy, and a lack of control over bowel and bladder function. Frequently, the dying depend on others for activities of daily life, a state that challenges those with an independent nature. Rarely is one prepared for the experience of being a MICU patient; movies, books, and TV shows tend to avoid graphic depictions of the critically ill.

Feelings associated with a loss of autonomy and dignity, with disfigurement, and with being a burden to loved ones are prevalent in the MICU. Moreover, not every MICU patient (or for that matter the loved ones of a MICU patient) has the time (or capacity) to cope with critical illness. The stages of coping with terminal illness (i.e., denial, anger, bargaining, depression, and acceptance) as enumerated by Elizabeth Kubler-Ross, in her classic book, "On Death and Dying," are not always dealt with in a specific order. Some individuals never get past denial; others never progress beyond anger. Others become morose and despondent, while still others, with the benefit of faith, appear more accepting. When critical illness strikes swiftly, adjustment is the most trying. But, grief, even when anticipated, is not easy to bear. Desperate measures may be invoked when death is imminent; some patients fight for life till the last breath is taken, and in this spirit, want anything and everything done that has any chance of facilitating relief or cure. Others, particularly those patients more accepting of the inevitability of death, and who have lived with illness for a long time, accept death and the comfort it can bring.

Often, the trajectory of illness is clear, which enables patients, family members, and staff time to say appropriate farewells. At these times, one attempts to have the patient be pain-free, and able to communicate effectively (in both a nonverbal manner, e.g., with reassuring touch, and with the ability to listen and to encourage expression of thoughts and feelings).

No doubt, repeated brushes with death threaten the physician's own equanimity, and can create a sense of loss. Some physicians defend themselves from the hardships of death by minimizing their own discomfort. They avoid involvement, use gallows humor, become mechanistic and overly intellectualized, talk at patients rather than listen to them, or are overly optimistic. Disappointment develops from not being able to save someone, and resentment is not far behind. While many criticize physicians for callousness and ineptitude, one should also consider that physicians are human; everyone has some difficulty facing death and communicating with the dying.

Theodore A. Stern, M.D.

May, 1984

I would hope and pray that in this long month I have helped at least one family to come to grips with the loss of a loved one; have dampened the horror/fright of the enveloping lights and buzzers in the mind of one critically ill old person fallen victim to our technological "marvels." If I have done this, my month wasn't wasted.

September, 1993

We did have one true save this month. She was a 42-year-old who came in with progressive shortness of breath, and was **intubated for** over a week with progressive **ARDS**. We sent every known test, all were negative. She did what people do and she got better on her own, and we did our part by avoiding … **iatrogenesis**. It seems so ironic that this was our only save as she was a drug addict who turned out to be quite unpleasant post-extubation. So it goes.

When we're here on Bigelow 9, we're generally way too busy to comprehend what transpires. Each pronounced patient is a tragedy to the friends/family who have been around them for all their life. We carry on, calling the **White desk** and filling out death certificates. We rarely have the time to comprehend what transpires here. It always seems more right when this process happens smoothly, without the dreaded "**dog shows.**" When the ball starts rolling, it is often difficult to break.

March, 1993

Your MICU experiences never die--they just become progressively more bizarre. Last month, on the **Bigelow**, I misplaced my stack of 3X5 patient cards, and looked everywhere for them, to no avail. I then encountered none other than Ms. Q, the woman with a **pH**

of 6.48 whom I admitted as an intern, now **status-post bilateral BKA**'s and admitted to another team, in her wheelchair in the hallway, flipping through my cards! Apparently heroin-free for two months. . .

January, 1986

SAR: "Mrs. X's renal function is improving." (She has rectal cancer with **ureteral obstruction)**.
Attending: "Good!"
SAR: "What's good about it?"
Attending: "She'll be able to take part in the decision of how she'll die."

In the midst of caring for critically ill individuals, residents search for the silver lining. While often said tongue-in-cheek, comments often reflect a desire to preserve patient autonomy for decision-making.

November, 1984

Regarding a 20-year-old **Walpole** inmate status-post drug overdose (suicide attempt):
JAR: "He may be very angry with us for saving his life."
SAR: "That's true, but he has the rest of his life to kill himself."

June, 1996

After 68 days at Mass. General, 56 of them in our ICU, Mrs. H passed away yesterday, with family at her bedside. Mrs. H had been full-go despite her critical illness and showed us the will to live, which was truly amazing. To have survived this long, she managed to see the birth of her grandchild and tell the new mother that she loved her, something that she had never done in the past.

April, 1991

I got to see a lot in the past 31 days, but a few cases stand out: I got to meet a nice older woman, walking and talking (rare in the MICU). She had a stream of family members in and out. They were worried about Grandma... She was smiling through the night, until she woke at 5:00 in the morning with the sense of impending doom. I got to know that look well. Right before our eyes, she lost her blood pressure. She was **DNR** by previous wishes. All we could do was stand by her bedside and hold her hand as her heart slowly stopped beating and she drifted off. No morphine drips, no withdrawal of support. She just died naturally, and we let her. Although hers was an unexpected death, we knew that she had a recent **MI**, and she wasn't a well person by any means. It struck me as not a bad way to go.

February, 1984

"In the end, I think she just died of entropy."

Dr. L (Attending), describing the demise of Ms. R, a 30-year-old woman with **cystic fibrosis**, who passed away at 4:30 this morning. He had known her for ten years and has been in the MICU since midnight for the 2nd night in a row. She could not survive until her lung transplant this Friday.

March, 1995

I just called another patient's daughter to tell her: "Your mother looks worse, you may want to come spend time with her."

"Do you mean my mother is going to die?"

It is hard not to feel a certain amount of responsibility of culpability in making such a phone call. Much easier to say: "She's doing well," and see them smile, than to see the horror and the dread.

My father still remembers, 30 years later, the words used by the doctor on the night my grandfather died.

December, 1984

The JAR and SAR were discussing a 27-year-old woman in a **neurovegetative** state for 22 days without any change in her neurologic status. The patient's father asked if there was permanent brain damage; The JAR explained that the chances of coming out of this state are 1 in 100,000. In a discussion about this the SAR replied, "You told him what!!?? You are such a pessimist."
The JAR asked, "What would you have told him?"
SAR: "1 in 1,000."

February, 1998

JAR to Dr. W: "Hey W--did you already pronounce Mr. O dead? I'd just as soon not repeat your work."
SAR: "That's okay. We needed a second opinion."

May, 1995

Dr. C (trying to figure out the best way to let the family know their loved one has passed away). "There's some good news, and some bad news. The good news is the bleeding has stopped. . ."

Gallows' humor, a type of humor intended to unearth the dark side of a terrible situation without feeling the emotional distress associated with that situation, is rampant in ICUs. Although this type of humor often is perceived as outrageous and insensitive, it acts as a defense against horror.

April, 1988

Tonight, a daughter requested I talk to her father about the futility of her mother's care--dense left stroke, severe **COPD**. No progress after hours of conversation. I tried hard to get him to understand we should not unnecessarily prolong her suffering and tried for a **DNR** status, i.e., don't **shock**. He is now very angry, and the rest of the family is upset. How could I have handled it better? Will I ever know? The MICU goes on . . .

February, 1984

Its raining and gray sky kicks up a little lump of loneliness. Sometimes it would be nice to go home with slippered feet, robe, and puff up a pipe. I'm not sure I've got any pipe cleaners guess I'll obsess about it. I think I left them under that moth-eaten sweater I stuck in the drawer in back of the closet. Now which closet was that, perhaps I'm losing it. This fear of aging deteriorating loss. It's kind of like the back pain of yesterday's picnic reminding you of the cost and loss of years and time to unwind out of this bind.

Hey man, toughen up, what is this sloppy sentiment? You're immortal. Or you've bought a little piece of the rock, I mean down the south shore. One of those plots with a headstone? No I mean a love-nest of a cottage. I'll go there with my honey and while away the hours with some castles made of sand.

May, 1987

Mr. B, a 30-year-old man with **ITP**, HIV, continuing to bleed overnight from his abdominal wound, despite the efforts of the intern and myself. He was 7 liters **TBB** positive, still bleeding, and very scared as he knew, as we did, that the end was near. It was way too overwhelming to contemplate this patient's thoughts. He was totally aware of his imminent death, while **intubated**, with wide eyes and alert, despite morphine going at 20 **cc** per hour. He is too young, too alert, too **coagulopathic**, breathing too much. We can't save him and yet, so many others who can't mentate remain among us.

March, 1980

We have two **status-post cardiac arrest anoxics** ventilating away right now. Between them, they can't muster a decent run of **EEG delta waves**—much less a sentient response. They will die soon. Tonight—now—if it weren't for us—we stand between them and peace—we stand between their families and a new, though perhaps sadder and more impoverished life. We prevent tomorrow from coming sooner and compel these unfortunate souls and their families to live in a ghostly limbo—an uncertain purgatory with the question being not heaven or hell—but hell—when? And why do we do this? Because we are unsure? Because we in medicine have decided that in matters of life and death....we must have no doubt? So we operate at the margins....

October, 1984

Said by the attending at **visit** rounds: "Look guys, just because he doesn't have a family and plays checkers all day doesn't mean we have a right to let him go 5 years before he's supposed to." (Speaking about an 84-year-old man with **aortic stenosis**.)

November, 1998

SAR: "T -- How do heart transplant patients regulate their heart rates?" Intern: "I dunno. . . it's a miracle the damn things work at all."

May, 1984

"I think we're fighting nature here."

Said by the attending in reference to Mr. A while he was in **VT** on **Xylo**, **Bretylium**, and **Pronestyl**, and on **Levo**, **Dopa**, **Isuprel**, and **Neo** to keep his systolic blood pressure about 60.

January, 1986

The intern, describing an 80-year-old Viennese cellist with **sick sinus syndrome:** "It's interesting, she escaped from Austria in the 1930s!" Attending: "The question is will she escape from **Bigelow 8**?"

December 25, 1990

Christmas Day in the MICU, and the team is discussing the construction materials used to make coffins . . . The JAR (about an unfortunate 60-year-old man with metastatic cancer, **sepsis**, renal failure, whose family wants him to die, but his oncologist isn't quite finished **cheeching**: "Mr. L needs a steel-lined coffin to keep his doctor out."

Correlary to above: The SAR (about a 97-year-old woman, demented, **septic**, **vented** (for the 90th time) who is actually doing well): "And Mrs. D needs a steel coffin to keep her in." Merry Christmas!

January, 1999

One of the youngest, and seemingly, the most normal patient on our service was patient A. We first met her as a **primary pulmonary hypertension** patient who was here to get her medications adjusted, and maybe get evaluated for a lung transplant. The books say it's a bad disease and these patients can get really sick really fast. However, it's hard to remember that when this normal, healthy young woman is seen working on her thesis while sitting in bed, covered in sheets she brought from home. We would wave to her as she pushed her IV pole around the unit--"this is not a MICU player," we would say on rounds. Morning pre-rounds would be spent talking about her dogs (she had a calendar made with pictures of her three dogs). She even took a "field trip" downstairs to see them one day.

Then the problems came--slowly at first. A little more **heart failure**, trouble adjusting her medications. Then, one day, in the morning, we found her, blood all over, and **aphasic**. She had bled into her head. It was a quick reminder that she wasn't a well person. Her problems multiplied. . . The team was demoralized--we felt that our healthiest patient was **iatrogenized** into one of the sickest.

But she recovered--she regained her faculties, her headache got better, her bleeding stopped. She was almost a save. Then--she had a **VT/VF arrest** refractory to **cardioversion** and the **code** was called at 6:00 AM. The patient's family and attending were notified.

The team was devastated. I was exhausted. We had essentially been coding another patient for the past 24 hours straight and we lost patient A on top of that. For most it was an emotional time. We had worked hard on her case, gotten close to her personally. Her loss is one that we all took to heart. But for me, I didn't feel it at all--too little sleep, too much work, too many responsibilities. I was totally numb. It was only after the event--after a decent night's sleep, a good meal, a shower--that I could feel human again--and thereby start to feel for her as well.

August, 1995

Mrs. P died yesterday. Her mother, who had made the decision to pull back, and has been by her side every day of her course, can now rest and mourn. I cannot even begin to imagine what it must be like to mourn for a child. But as I await the birth of my first--I have a sense that there could be nothing worse.

May, 1985

Dr. S, quoting a congressman of the U.S. House of Representatives during hearing regarding federal funding of health insurance: "Death is cheap, and even cheaper when it occurs early in life."

This statement is striking. While technically correct, that death in a young person consumes fewer healthcare dollars, the human aspects are ignored. When economics are broached in the ICU, a hidden conflict is usually present. Numbers easily replace the human element and protect the discussants from anger and loss.

November, 1984

To share one of the unpleasant ICU experiences—telling a close friend with an Italian-speaking mother that their father/husband is "**brain dead**" when they can see full well that his breathing and heart will stop only when I turn off the **vent**.

--wanting to say that it is indecent to breath for someone who has been dead for 4 days when they ask, "What's the rush?"

--thinking about turning off the respirator when they leave the room and knowing you can't in good conscience (but "legally" you could).

--hoping that his heart will stop but knowing that it won't. Wishing someone else had turned off the respirator this morning.

--agreeing to wait until the whole family has been notified of his "death"—and hearing them all say alternatively, "He doesn't look any different" or "Why did you prolong this pain for his wife if you knew he was dead?"

May, 1986

On rounds this morning, we were discussing a story of Isaac Beshevis Singer's—in which a dying man "sells" his sins to a poor schlimazel, to obtain a country dream home. This dying man was "an upstanding community leader," thought by many, including the schlimazel, to have few sins to his record. But later, when he went to heaven's gate... well....

In this vein, Dr. W asked about possibly purchasing sins from some of our patients. But he pointed out—"One does not know for sure the sins of someone **lined**, **tubed**, **vented**." I guess knowing a patient's **wedge** is not enough.

June, 1984

10:00 on a **swing** night. It's days like today that I just don't feel it anymore. I guess that's a bad thing to write in the "red" book. I just want to be home. Beam me home, Scotty.

It's funny. I loved the ICU as an intern, my favorite place. I also thought, "The ICU JAR is a great job." I guess so. Seems more political now, more beds, White 8, nurses...and "would you just talk to the family about status." The ICU is the only place where having status is bad for you. Mr. T, nice man, tough, denies his **ejection fraction of 11%** (tough to deny that). Improving a little on **dobutamine**, **captopril**, **IV TNG**, **bumex**, kitchen sink. Family having a hard time coming to grips with his illness, (he worked up to the day of his **MI**) tries to understand. The nurse mentions on rounds, "Where are we going here, we need a status." I see the attending speaking with Mr. T, then Mr. T and wife, then just the wife, off and on all day as the nurse leaves at 5 p.m. Later tonight while I'm putting in an **A-line** I hear of a transfer from the emergency department and the need to rearrange beds. A nurse says, "....oh move the **DNR** in 27, he's no work."

Mr. T has attained a "status." Tomorrow will be better.

January, 1992

There is a party atmosphere in the visitor's lounge. A **lymphoma** patient's family is reminiscing about their relative's life and preparing for his death. His wife is holding court and thanking everyone for coming. When she is walking in circles, unable to decide what to do… her sons bicker and tell her to decide one way or the other, whether or not to go home. She thinks "If I go home, will he die?… If I stay will he die? In feeble resolve she enters the unit to say goodbye - only to be told "we're not ready for you now." She dissolves in her powerlessness.

There is a party atmosphere in the unit. The staff is chatty, facile, and efficient. We do not dissolve in our powerlessness. We have little resolve and cannot reminisce.

October, 1985

For some of the patients in the unit the following lines resonate:
"Just want to have, a little place to die
And a friend or two I love at hand."—The Grateful Dead.

A short and sweet philosophy that often is not achieved.

October, 1997

Plenty of people have come through the MICU this month that have been patched up and sent back to the floor. Yet, it strikes me that in the Saves column, after 59 admissions and only 12 deaths, they only tally two. There are no formal criteria for what a save entails, but clearly, our attitude is that unless someone is on death's door and has very little chance for survival, and is very young, they don't count. We don't give ourselves enough credit for the people we've helped, and only credit a "save" when there is an incredibly small chance for one in the first place.

The perfectionist attitude is no doubt at the center/route of how down we were about one particular "**Allen Street**" entry, who, even if we had got her to transplant safely, she would not have counted as a "save."

It's a hard way to be be--to not give yourself credit for victories, however small, and to torture yourself about outcomes you had absolutely no control over at any time.

It is also interesting to me how much more down you can get in response to death than you seem to get up when you save life.

Ours is not an easy job. Until next year,

In the conference room at the rear of the MICU, in which the house-staff meet each morning and evening for sign-in/out rounds, a chalk-board hangs at one end of a long table. Each month, the new team assiduously records the month's happenings, in column format, in terms of numbers of admissions, deaths, saves, ethical saves (meaning, a person who, in the team's opinion, should be allowed to die, is allowed to die), and other categories.

March, 1990

"I did not die, yet nothing of life remained." --Dante.

June, 1980

The sun is born and dies and comes again.
The moon is born and dies and comes again.
The stars are born and die and come again.
Man is born and dies and does not come again.

December, 1987

Dr. R referring to **DNR** patient who is about to **extubated**: "He no fly... he die."

February, 1983

"You can't get out of life alive."

November, 1981

Of course, it's a gray area—that's why we have a gray solution.

One-liners, brief quotes, and attempts at philosophy punctuate the daily grind.

December 24, 1990

AKA: "It's a wonderful unit." Just remember, every time you start a morphine drip, an angel gets its wings....

June, 1993

A Patient Note:
"I don't want to hear, 'Hang in there'! I have been here since the 14th. I want it out, and call my husband with the results."

Stages of Death--Last Stage--Acceptance:
This note is written by a 53-year-old woman with **Scleroderma Lung**, who was enrolled for lung transplant three years earlier, and came here for a **catheterization**, after which she dropped her **O2 Sats**. She was **intubated**. On day #5, the JAR and I went to see her in the morning. She wrote the note after we said, "Hang in there, Mrs. X." The patient

demanded that we take the tube out, she understood the outcome, including death, and had discussed it with her husband and her son. The tube was pulled out after rounds. Gradually, she became **hypoxic** and **hypercarbic**. I went to see her every 30 minutes.

She appeared comfortable, facing death with a smile. She passed away at 7:15 a.m., her family was at her bedside. I was very emotional after that whole experience. It was an ethical save. She had a chronic disease and was comfortable with death, leaving a loving husband and son behind. May God bless her soul.

CHAPTER FIVE:

Patients and Families

Despite our methodical natures, or our measured, critical thinking, the choices we make at life's crossroads often eschew science. That is, notwithstanding the efforts we go through to carefully balance the advantages and downsides to important decisions, in the end we let emotions guide us, and work backwards to justify ourselves rationally.

My first day of residency in Boston, we sat in a conference room that smelled vaguely of Indian food, the remnant of lunches from past noon conferences. We were handed our rotations for the next year, the schedule that would determine whether we would be able to join our families for Thanksgiving, go out to parties on New Year's Eve, or even wake when our bodies told us to on a given Sunday morning. I was focused more on where I would have to report the next morning: to the MICU, or Deathstar, as the older residents liked to call it. I had never rotated through a MICU as a medical student, and thus was completely unfamiliar with how to manage these critically ill bodies masquerading as sentient human beings. And I was on-call the first night.

This would turn into the longest day of my life. I met my junior resident, Dave, the person who would share my call nights, at 7 a.m., and he helped me make it through rounds with the MICU staff, fellow, senior resident, two other junior residents, and two other interns. To put it more plainly, he did all the work of writing notes, making decisions about patients, and placing invasive lines, while I ran errands for him, and was thrilled when I could successfully locate an X-ray in the catacombs of the radiology department.

As night fell, we rounded out, during which the other intern-junior pairs told us about their patients, and then took their leave, a scene straight out of a World War II movie, in which the company is forced to abandon the two guys whose legs were shot up, leaving them with a certain amount of ammunition to fend off the advancing Germans. They always say goodbye and promise to come back to retrieve the guys the next morning – if they survive the night, which everyone knows is highly unlikely.

Among the usual medical disasters we would care for that night – the old people with consuming pneumonias, the patients with dissecting aortas, or hearts that beat at one-tenth their usual capacity – was a woman, a pediatrician from a nearby hospital, who had widely metastatic ovarian cancer and whose lungs were filling with fluid. Initially, she was to be intubated and placed on a respirator, but she changed her mind, deciding instead to live her last hours breathing air on her own, unassisted. She was in her early 40s, and her appearance in our unit had consumed our team's emotions that day. It didn't help matters when her son and daughter, ages 10 and 8, came in to say goodbye to her in the evening – what we all knew would be the last time they would see her. Each of us in turn, doctors and nurses, sought refuge off the main floor to check the hitch in our breathing, or outright cry in private.

Her husband escorted their children away and returned a couple of hours later with her best friend, now carrying a CVS bag. As I was doing my rounds, checking vitals on patients to dutifully report back to Dave, I glanced in her room, and saw her husband standing, hunched over her bed, holding a clipboard as she wrote something. I made it back to our conference room.

"Hey Dave, what's going on in there?" I asked, gesturing to her room. By this point of the day, I had proven myself to be so utterly helpless, I no longer even worried about asking Dave completely idiotic questions. He was my life-line, my only source of truth. If I had even time to go to the bathroom, I probably would have needed his assistance with that, too. He looked at me blandly, but without prejudice.

"She's writing out cards."

"3 x 5 cards?" I asked? I had a pocket full of them, each with a different patient's information written. The only cards I could picture.

"No, birthday, holiday cards, those types."

Birthday, holiday cards, graduation cards, cards for every occasion she could imagine. Cards for bar and bat mitzvahs. Cards for Halloween. Cards for the next 10 years for her son and daughter. Cards so she could be a part of their lives. Cards because she was so proud of them. Cards so she could live those years with them over the course of her last night on earth. Cards so they would never forget her.

I was up all night, caring for others, and watching her stay up all night, writing, sometimes her husband holding the clipboard, sometimes her friend. The sun rose over the Charles River, she finished, and as her breathing became more labored, she asked that her morphine dose be increased.

Over a decade has passed, and I still think about her all the time. I wonder if I would do the same for my children, now that I have them, or how I would deal with this cache of missives from another world, if I were her husband. I also think of her son and daughter – did they look forward to getting these cards throughout the year, or dread them? Did they save them? As a parent, I would hope so. But maybe her uncertain handwriting during her final hours reminded her kids of the time when she was sick, so they rejected the cards for earlier, happier memories.

I became an oncologist. Ironically, years later, Dave himself developed cancer, and called me for help. I can provide perfectly rational reasons for my career choice, including the fascinating pathobiology of the diseases, the opportunities for translational research, or the prospects for conducting clinical trials of novel agents. But really, it's to have even a glancing connection to people who face these terrible diseases with dignity, and in so doing, give value to the lives of everyone around them. It's because of that woman, who wanted to have a say after her death.

Mikkael Sekeres, M.D., M.S.
(Reprinted from *Journal of Clinical Oncology* 2010;28:5348-9.)

January, 1985

Delirious patient to team: "No man! Don't do that (**IV** placement). I'll give you all jobs at $7.50 an hour."
Attending: "This guy could be the stuff of which legends are made."

June, 1987

SAR: "I don't know why we consider her incompetent. She walks, talks, eats—it's not like she's jumping in front of cars or out of windows."
JAR: "Well, she did light her hair on fire."
SAR: "Oh....that was a mistake."

May, 1986

The patient admitted for complaints of shortness of breath eventually requiring **intubation**. Apparently he had two dogs to which he was allergic. His allergies had become so severe that the day of admission he had put them to sleep. "Not soon enough."

May, 1987

Mr. B, a patient who presented with an **inferior wall MI** after walking his pit bull, has post-**MI** pain, went to **cath**, has terrible **coronary artery disease**, and needs a **CABG**.
Attending: "We think you need bypass surgery."
Mr. B: "Can't I just get rid of the dog and take it easy?"

December, 1992

Daughter of a brain-dead patient who was unwilling to let her mother go, offers "to do" our attending in return for not pulling the plug.

When confronted with impending death, it is common for patients or their families to offer to make a "deal with the devil" in exchange for tranquillity or health. Rarely do such deals lead to their intended result.

February, 1996

So often I feel we strip people of their dignity and peace, and yet, a few moments shine through. Mr. X, facing death after a long hospital course with lymphoma, renal failure, saying, "It's okay. I know you can't save me. Tell my family not to cry." Watching families come to grips with the loss of their loved ones always leaves an ache in my heart. So often we "rearrange the deck chairs on the Titanic," but forget to mourn the sinking ship. I hope the hot sun and open canyons of Arizona renew my spirits. I can't leave without a final goodbye to Mr. V All month I tried, kept hoping he'd get better. I think I've come to see him as the Eeyore that sits near his bed. Just like the story, we never could get that tail pinned back on. May you find peace!

October 31, 1998

So perverse, it must be the MICU:
Mrs. C, a lady with endstage lung disease and **change in mental status**, is visited by a relative who brings her a mechanized stuffed crow which, when a button is pressed, cries out: "Caw! Caw! Caw! Beware, the end is near!"
Looks like our senior just lost his job to a battery-operated crow. . .

Instead of a raven quoting, "Nevermore," the crow cawed that the end was near. Notice how a member of the team relegates the senior's job to that of Angel of Death.

July, 1986

A 380-pound man (also rumored to be a hit man) said to the intern, as he was placing an **A-line**: "You get two tries, the third shot is mine."

The deal-making continues, only now with a different slant. Deals are suggested as a way to exert control over one's illness. At times, a threat to the safety of physicians is as real as the danger to patients.

March, 1995

Ms. B, a 57-year-old, **intubated**, but very alert and communicative patient, after approximately 30 **arterial line** attempts by the JAR and me one evening, wrote a note to her daughter on the clipboard: "If I had had a gun last night, there would have been a couple of dead doctors!" Needless to say, we were not present when she was **extubated**!"

November, 1998

Dr. R, after explaining to the patient with **primary pulmonary hypertension**, that the risk of **calcium-channel blockers** includes death and she needs to sign informed consent: "Well, I'll sign that form but my father will still come after you."
We wonder how many other fathers have come after Dr. R…

As a defense against threats, humor is employed; the specter of prior sexual relationships and solutions eases the tension. "Informed consent" indicates that a patient gives permission to receive a medication or have a procedure performed after having the risks and benefits of that medication or procedure explained in simple terms.

June, 1995

After seeing an **arrhythmia** on the monitor, an eager JAR comes to the rescue and thumps the chest of an awake Mr. I, who replies: "That's not very nice!"

December, 1988

Dr. L innocently walking through the ICU one day notices a frail 75-year-old woman who suddenly develops **VT** without loss of consciousness. L rushes into the room and delivers a **precordial thump**. The woman is successfully converted to **normal sinus rhythm**. Her first words: "All I wanted was the bedpan, and she hit me!!"

April, 1987

Recounted by the attending, about the old **Bulfinch ICU**. A new patient was transferred into the room and an old patient was overheard telling the new patient, "You hear that beep, beep, beep overhead?"
"Yeah."
"Well if you stop hearing that beep, beep, beep...you'd better start saying beep, beep, beep...'cause otherwise they'll all coming running in and beat on your chest."

July, 1986

The SAR, chatting with a **cachectic** 76-year-old woman:
SAR: "I see you're wearing lipstick today."
Patient: "Yes...would you like to taste it?"

Confusion in the ICU takes many forms, though some would like to believe that this was just another deal.

July, 1986

Wow! What an amazing month. I've always been too intimidated to write in this book, but the experience here this time around leaves me no choice. Here is a review of some of my most difficult moments. . .

--Having to **code** Patient N, a 37-year-old woman with a huge **MI**, after making a decision to pull her **IABP**, joking with her moments before she arrested, coding for 1 ½ hours with four cardiologists and the bedside **IABP** insertion, and being unable to bring her back--that was defeat, and nothing prepares you for that. (Giving up is easy in comparison to trying your hardest and still failing).

--Having to watch our favorite patient, Mrs. M, after dying of **VF**, being wheeled out on a stretcher, covered with a sheet, during the rounds she used to cheer up so much with her smile (lipstick-laden) and funny stories. . .

In spite of and even particularly because of, these difficult moments, this has been an excellent month for me. I've learned a lot about life/death/medicine/hope/leadership/teamwork/compassion/disappointment. . . you name it, it's here. All you need is enough support and sense of humor to allow you to get close enough to what's going on. I thank everyone on my team.

February, 1997

Mr. H, an 84-year-old with improving **mental status**.
Nurse: "Do you know who the president is?"
Mr. H: "Well, I know it's not Lincoln!"

January, 1999

Regarding a patient with **mental status exam** the morning after admission performed by the attending:
"What's the date?"

"January 1999."
"Where are you?"
"In the hospital."
"Who's the president?"
"Garibaldi."
"Garibaldi?"
"Oh, that's Italy, not here."

Given recent impeachment proceedings, this answer may have been understandable. However, the president of Italy is actually Scarpoli, and Garibaldi was a patriot famous in the 1800s.

Interestingly, at the time the physicians and nurses in the room did not know that Garibaldi was not the president of Italy, either. For housestaff and for some patients, keeping track of recent information is hampered by the isolation of the ICU. A variety of simplistic questions of orientation are part and parcel of the mental status examination.

June, 1996

On Morning Rounds:
"So, Mr. B (a quite confused alcoholic man) do you know where you are?"
"Up the fat lady's ass."
"Close. . ."

November, 1991

My month here has taught me that medicine is an art. After 3 years at the MGH, we as residents are well tuned to deal medically with **arrhythmias**, **hypotension**, and the like. But in the setting of the ICU where patients often role in with irreversible **multi-system organ failure**, the goal for hospitalization is in such cases not cure but care. As a senior in the ICU, I found myself spending much time comforting patients and caring for distraught members of the patients' families. "Should my 9-year-old, whose mother is gravely ill in the ICU, come to visit?" "What can I say to my father who is dying?" "Do you think my brother (on respirator for **ARDS**) will make it?" "Is he in pain?" As patients slip deeper into the gray zone between life and death, I often found myself asking: "Are we buying life or prolonging death?" "What is 'quality of life' for this patient?" And "what would I do if this patient were my own family?" These are truly difficult questions that must be addressed, not simply by counting the number of irreversible organ system failures and tallying prognoses, but also by counting on family members to express what the patient would want were he/she able to speak for themselves. There is no science that can quantitate what "life force/energy" (in far eastern medicine called "Jing" and "Qi") still ebbs in a patient. Thus I realize how much art is in the practice of medicine.

March, 1996

Mr. L, a near drowning patient, after trying to rescue two other people, says to the team prior to his exam: "Pardon the sewage breath."

Many houseofficers believe that they employ heroic measures to save critically ill patients. But in their own right, patients' heroic efforts may have lead to their ICU admission. Their altruism is a touching part of their character.

July, 1990

The JAR was called in to see a patient for chest pain. After spending what seemed like hours trying to relieve the chest pain with morphine, **IV TNG**, **IV Inderal**, and **heparin**, the JAR looks up at the TV to find a porno movie on. He writes in the orders: 1. **DC** Showtime. 2. Stat surgery consult for a **bilateral orchiectomy**.

December, 1995

Mr. R, a 400-lb. **COPD-er**, blew himself up cooking on his gas stove while attached to his home oxygen. In the Burn Unit, he was **intubated** and transferred to the MICU. He was **extubated** today, after 4 days on the **vent** by the intern, with the Knicks--Pacers game playing in the background.
Intern: "How are you feeling Mr. R? Glad to have the tube out?"
Mr. R: "Get out of the way. I can't see the game."

Sometimes the priorities of the physicians are not the same as those of the patients.

March, 1986

Patient: "Ow, ow, ow, ow, ow, ow, ow, ow, ow, ow, ow, ow, ow, ow, ow, ow, ow."
Attending: "Does that hurt?"
Patient: "Sure it hurts. Otherwise I wouldn't be saying ow."

April, 1986

80-year-old woman with **complete heart block**, **heart rate of 28**: "Why do I need a pacemaker? I eat; I shit, I breathe."

July, 1998

In Mr. M's room, awakening from a long sleep:
JAR: "Mr. M, can you hear me?"
Mr. M: Nods yes.
JAR: "Are you in pain?"
Mr. M: Nods yes.
JAR: "Does your throat hurt?"
Mr. M: Nods yes.

JAR: "Does your chest hurt?"
Mr. M: Nods yes.
JAR: "Does your belly hurt?"
Mr. M: Nods Yes.
JAR (aside): "I guess he only says yes. Can you shake your head no?"
Mr. M: Does nothing.
JAR: "I guess there's no way to get him to say no."
SAR: "Mr. M, do you like the Yankees?"
Mr. M: Shakes his head no.

Mental status assessments sometimes require questions with high emotional tone. Denying an affinity for the Yankees penetrated even the near-comatose state of this Boston resident.

October, 1991

The team on rounds outside Mr. I's room beginning to discuss his prior events when Mr. I, who overheard the team, states: "Mr. I left! He was transferred!"

February, 1993

A patient was admitted for pneumonia. When questioned about his Penicillin allergy, his wife secretly told our critical care fellow, "Oh, he's not really allergic. They gave it to him once and it didn't work, so I tell everyone he's allergic."

October, 1985

A note rests on the soda-machine:

"Do not remove please. This machine owes me 30 cents."

(Signed: Mrs. N).

Deep thoughts from Mrs. N After only a few million dollars stay for her husband at the MGH ICU, Mrs. N, looking to find a bargain/rebate.

Patients often attempt to take medicine into their own hands and reestablish a sense of control. Sometimes the big picture is lost.

April, 1990

A rare slow day for the team--a Sunday. Lots of families around--notably, these 70-ish year-old parents of Mr. I He is a 41-year-old man transferred from an outside hospital "**big and yellow**" and bleeding out from an undefined source. His parents have decided (less than 36 hours after his transfer to Mass. General and his **intubation**) that they would like to pull back and let him die. So here I sit as this young man bleeds out and his parents (Pa in his wheelchair, Ma with her grey hair and spectacles) wait by his bedside. They don't speak to each other, cry, or even look at him--their son--who they have decided doesn't even want blood products. What spurs on their decision? When sons and daughters will keep their 90-year-old parents on vents 'til Kingdom comes? Somehow, I feel better if there were tears, or indecision or some manifestation of grief. Without these--their decision seems so cold, heartless--did he steal money from them for his alcoholic binges? Crash their car? Wreck their house? How little we know about all the elements which defacto go into such momentous decisions. Not that I disagree-- his death is near regardless of treatment. Something about how they sit impassively, and yes, almost impatiently, waiting for their son to die, chills me.

Sometimes physicians lose the big picture as well.

April, 1993

The intern, presenting a patient: "He was passed off to me as being completely **aphasic** but in fact, this is not true--he could say "mother fucker," with the best of them."

December, 1994

"Get this fucking machine off me." Mr. C, thanking the ICU team for his 3 weeks of vigilant care, and immediately after his successful **extubation**.

January, 1993

Commenting on a woman with **anoxic encephalopathy**, with a family that wants **a full court press**, who is now found to have **killer klebsiella** in her **sputum** and in her urine, the JAR comments:
"She's a **Petrie dish**."

Faced with multi-system organ failure and a terminal course, humor is used to take the edge off.

September, 1993

Dr. I, describing the psychiatric state of Mr. T, a 33-year-old man **status-post aortic valve** replacement and **aortic graft** placement, now with an **embolic stroke** and requiring another heart surgery:
"If he's not depressed, then he's not paying attention to what's going on."

February, 1988

Regarding a patient who drinks two to three quarts of alcohol per day, smokes five to six packs per day:
JAR #1: "How does he have time to do both?"
JAR #2: "He's a disciplined guy."

June, 1994

When talking with the family of a man with alcoholic **hepatic encephalopathy**, they informed me that he drinks 7-9 glasses of whiskey a day for 30 years. In reiterating the history, I said: "His dad has been an alcoholic for 30 years." The family (son) states: "Let's not call him an alcoholic. Let's just say he has a high tolerance."

Many family members, having lived with substance use and abuse for years, deny what is obvious to others and conspire with the user to avoid treatment.

March, 1992

The attending, in regards to a former **IVDA**, burglar, **status- post** imprisonment, now bleeding profusely from esophageal **varices**, "Did he ever have a meaningful life?"

August, 1997

Attending Rounds, HMS presenting: "The patient took a whole bottle of **Loxapine** in a suicide attempt and then called the **EMTs**."
The attending: "Another mixed message."

July, 1994

On a.m. Rounds, while discussing Ms. L, a heroin addict admitted post-overdose, Dr. E explained how every addict (according to the patient's fiancé) knows **CPR**: "They have performed CPR on one another several times after their multiple overdoses."
The SAR's response: "Oh, what did they say--Annie, Annie, can I have the rest of your bags?"

All physicians are required to take American Red Cross Basic Lifesaving and Advanced Lifesaving courses. In the Basic Lifesaving course, participants are taught the "ABCs" (Assess a person to make sure she has an open Airway, that she is Breathing, and that she has a working Circulatory system – a pulse). While "evaluating" the dummy victim, named "Annie," during the Red Cross class, participants are taught to shout at her, "Annie, Annie, can you hear me??!!" This is an exercise in determining a victim's alertness and ability to speak and thereby breathe.

July, 1981

Wife of overdose patient (previous overdose history) decided this time he needed to come to the hospital because he did not respond when she placed his testicles in cold water.

October, 1991

Just another case of a close, caring, intimate relationship. Mr. N, **status-post VF arrest**..."He lives with his girlfriend/common law wife. She thought he didn't look quite right earlier in the day but she went shopping anyway. When she returned he was unresponsive on the bed. She waited a few minutes and then called 911 and then sat and watched. 15 minutes later the **EMT**s arrived. After **intubating** the patient and performing **ACLS**...the EMTs turned to the girlfriend and told her it was time to go to the hospital. Her response was, "I can't right now I have to feed the dogs."

Addendum to Mr. N above—the common-law wife gave us the phone number of the sister—it rang up a pay phone on a street corner, answered by a passerby who knew no such person. Some people have all the luck.

November, 1992

At dinner, the JAR returns to the conference room after answering the seventh page from his psychotic alcoholic patient: "He (the patient) is now saying that he is threatening to kill himself by chopping both hands off with an ax."
HMS: "Cheer up, T, that's impossible. You can only chop off one hand."

February, 1991

A patient came to the MICU billed as a suicide attempt, **intubated** with a negative **toxicology screen**, despite finding the patient in vomit with empty **Klonopin** and **Valproate** bottles. Suicide note states: "Tell those bitches that I am leaving." The next morning the patient is awake and "yelling "to get the **tube** out. He is **extubated** and the SAR attempts to fill in the gaps in our history.
SAR: "Why did you try to kill yourself?"
Patient: "What the Hell are you talking about?"
SAR: "We found your suicide note."
Patient: "Suicide note? I was just moving to Cambridge. I didn't want my sisters to be worried."
SAR: "But what about the empty Valproate, and Klonopin bottles?"

Patient: "I ran out of pills and probably had a seizure!"
Oops!

March, 1987

Dr. I: "I got the history from the patient's wife who, well...the butter slipped off the noodle a long time ago."

January, 1996

The intern, in reference to Mr. O, a 34-year-old drug user, not responding to commands: "He's not the sharpest hoe in the shed, you know." Nurse, in response: "Yeah, but he kind of blunted his own instruments, didn't he. . ."

Ninety percent of successfully diagnosing and treating an illness depends on an accurate patient history, or retelling of events that led up to the illness. When the history is inaccurate and cannot be obtained directly from a patient, impressions and treatment can be misguided or delayed. The residents' frustration aimed at the family members is almost palpable.

August, 1997

After nearly 2 months of being **vented**, Mr. R says, using his talking **trach.**, "I want a beer," then becomes confused again.

June, 1984

Discussion with a patient ambulating **status-post MI** on **White 8**.
Patient: "Well, how long doc?"
ICU Team: "Oh about 5 days."
Patient: "You mean I'm going to die on Monday???"

November, 1993

The SAR today gravely informed the wife of a 70-year-old massively obese man with critical **AS**, **CHF**, and **sepsis**, that he had taken a turn for the worse and was now **intubated** and was now on **pressors**. Understandably, she took the news hard.

The two of them walked down the Unit and stopped opposite the patient's room, where Mr. B was lying intubated, agitated, and nearly naked with **EKG leads** strewn across his chest; there was abundant debris scattered about the room, remnants of the near **code** that had just ensued.

However, Mrs. B turned and stared into the adjacent room of Mr. S, a long-term **ARDS** patient, who was freshly shaved and washed and had a new set of johnnies and was lying peacefully and comfortably. She said, "Oh my God, that's not him, is it??!"

SAR: "No, no, no, he's doing fine," taking her arm hastily, leading her out the door.

When thinking is less than sharp, miscommunication and misinterpretation may complicate care. Life-long patterns of behavior often shine through the clouded thought. The patient asking for a beer probably was intubated as a consequence of alcoholism.

January, 1986

A 93-year-old patient who **presented** in **complete heart block** with a **heart rate of about 30** explained, "They're going to put in a permanent dressmaker."

February, 1991

At work rounds, the intern reporting about a new admission: a young man found acting bizarrely at a Grateful Dead concert.

"Patient claims he could breathe only when looking straight into my eyes."

Attending: "Oh, that's so romantic!"

Intern: "The patient was only partially oriented to self. He knew his first name but not his last name."

JAR, **running the issues**: "Okay, neurologically...he's a Deadhead."

The difficulty of managing a failing heart and a young man unable to breathe cause reactions of sadness in physicians, which is dealt with by the turning of phrases and word play.

February, 1999

The intern, speaking of Ms. G, who has been **intubated** forever but still hasn't quite awakened from her sedation...

"**Neurology** found out she is able to communicate via telekinesis on today's **EEG**--she has a 6th sense."

May, 1994

Discussing Mr. D, a gentleman with a **locked-in state**, who communicated only by blinking, and who was found to have had a **respiratory arrest**:

JAR #1: "He may have **anoxic brain damage**."

JAR #2: "He may never blink again!?"

Once again, the tragedy of profound neurologic dysfunction and recuperation from burns is made acceptable by use of absurdity.

March, 1993

A patient with renal cell cancer, evaluated by the Optimal Care Committee, who reported: "His son called a tech a "fucking moron." We can assume he's upset."

April, 1991

Mr. Q, 55-year-old male **schizophrenic** veteran with severe **coronary artery disease**, demands to smoke "like in the VA." He is on for a **cath** in the a.m. He is getting agitated. The SAR firmly believes that Mr. Q can be convinced to cooperate. A contract is made, the order is written: "patient may be accompanied to smoking lounge for one cigarette at 1:00, 5:00, 8:00 p.m." The interns, after accompanying patients to **CT scans**, etc., accompany Mr. Q out for a butt. The SAR escorts him at 8, and reports, "He is the most bizarre individual I've ever met." This impresses the team. Upon returning, Mr. Q announces that now he wants "a cigarette every hour all night."
"That's not in the contract!" says the SAR.
"I'm leaving," says Mr. Q
"Get me an **AMA** form!" The SAR is an idealist but also a realist.

September, 1991

A patient being observed in the unit for cardiac **tamponade**: "My doctor said it could be a virus or maybe stress. I do work with explosives, but that's nothing."

January, 1987

Mr. L has returned to the MICU for the eigth time in 7 months, and his seventh **intubation** during this time period. The last time he was intubated, the JAR joked to the patient as he was wheeled into the unit: "I have to go to the bathroom real bad, take your **ambu bag**." Mr. L **bagged** himself as he was wheeled into the room.

It is uncommon for patients in the ICU to be verbal, coherent, and helpful in their own care. When it does occur, it engenders likeability.

October, 1997

Littered papers on the table, scribbled words--"Let me die, please." Dated as if to make it legal. On the pretext of going to her room, I can't forget the 8 **angiocaths** reddened with her blood, dulled by her thick skin. Her weak hand then tried to tell me stop, please stop, please stop. I knew what she was saying, I think, but she wasn't quite human yet. Now, she's stronger--much stronger than me--and paralyzes me with her firmness.

"I'm sorry," I say to her. "I'm really sorry for all we have put you through, please forgive me." She looks at me with her wide opaque eyes, and lays her hand on mine, she comforts me. She mouths "thank you," and asks, "How long?" She's eager for the end now, like a bride--impatient. We have tried for an hour to convince her husband that she's depressed, that she can't make this decision, that you only live once, and she may return to some functional capacity--only go through dialysis 3 out of 7 days. He shifts uncomfortably, and then tells us quite clearly: "She never wanted this."

February, 1996

Dr. S, commenting on the ethical disaster Mr. Q, quadriplegic, multiply infected, intermittently communicative with eyes blinking, **in-house** for 6 months because his family believed that his suffering earned him a better place in his next life:
"Wow, he must be a rock star in Heaven by now!"

July, 1997

I remember talking with other students last year about how at the end of the fourth year, one gets frustrated at always needing a **co-sign**, never truly getting the trust of the nurses whenever you're doing an invasive procedure, etc. Right now, however, I feel occasional pangs of these frustrations but since the **match**, I have also been keenly aware of the safety net I now enjoy, as well as the vast amount of knowledge I do not know and will not know, even in July. I have to say that I have loved my time in the MICU this month, on call, with the JAR and intern. There have been times this month when I have laughed so hard I **aspirated** my coffee. There was also one night when patient A pulled out her **A-line** and the intern and I each tried that night to put it in without success. I think both he and I were on the brink of tears (although he probably won't admit to it). That weekend, I felt so depressed and frustrated for A, especially because, in the end, we had decided to manage her without the line, and we had put her through so much "torture" (her word). I prayed for her that Sunday night--okay, it sounds geeky--like something we talk about in **Ethics Rounds**--but I think, in our own way, we all were . . . Our greatest relief was when she did get better, and when I asked her about the A-line attempts, she did not remember them at all. How strange to take care of people with moods and personality and irritating habits, like pulling out their lines, and have it be that so much of our interaction with them is easily forgotten.

Goodbye team; goodbye Book. The next time you see me, I will be flying without a safety net.

June, 1992

Our role as doctors in the MICU gives us such a privileged advantage--we peer into some of the most intimate scenes of a person's life, simply by walking past the windows to their rooms. The images are haunting--patient B, six weeks **post-partum**, now awakens from a drug-induced coma, after **ECMO** for pneumonia, holding the child she gave birth to for the first time (still **trached** and **vented** with an **A-line** to boot); the distraught son who tearfully clenched his neurologically-devastated mother's hand and noted that, "I love her so much, she has worked so hard that she would not mind living this way (blind, quadriplegic, ventilation-dependent)", simply because he could not bear to say farewell; Mr. H--awake after 3 weeks of sedation, crying at the sight of his favorite things (his friends, chocolate pudding, his mother--whom he asked to sleep over so he would not feel afraid in his dark corner room); Mr. T, a 22-year-old with **ARDS** on **ECMO,** a boy who seemed merely an extension of a machine, a vent, mysteriously un-alive, despite our technological battle to save him.

The memories linger. The lessons live--grow. The MICU moves on. I have no doubt that our team, each and every member--is very different now, after a mere 31 days. We cherish these "snapshots," we treasure our view.

November, 1990

Scene: Mr. D's death bed. Family is gathered around in devoted vigil. Enter the JAR.
Mrs. D: (smiling) "Hey everybody. Who does she look exactly like (pointing to the JAR).
Family (chorus): "Yes, yes! (chants!). She really does!
Mrs. D: (still smiling) "You look exactly like the barmaid my son (Mr. D) had an affair with! You can see the way he stares at you?! You are making him so happy now. It's amazing!"
Family (chorus): "Yes, it's really nice. You look just like her!"
Nurse (to JAR): "I guess they found out about your night job."

December, 1990

The JAR, is called away from work rounds to deal with chest pain in a gentleman 2 days out from an **IMI**. She walks into the room to find the patient insisting on standing up to relieve his pain. The JAR and the ICU nurse convince the patient that this is not allowed and compromise on the patient rolling onto his side. A voluminous and malodorous sample of flatulence is released from the patient and "ta da," gone is the **5/10 chest pain**!

Now the patient is having chest pain again and is **hypotensive**, in **trendelenberg**. The JAR enters the room: "How's your gas?" she inquires. "Oh, it's coming out the right end now," replies the patient.

April, 1985

Who said **visit** rounds aren't therapeutic?

The attending, pressing on patient's **costochondral junctions** looking for chest wall pain: "Does this hurt?"
Patient: "No I'm enjoying it! Thanks for the rubdown!"

July, 1985

SAR (to elderly, hallucinatory lady with diabetes, **chronic renal failure**, depression): "Do you remember your doctor, Dr. G?"
Patient: "Ooohhhh...oooo...aaaahh!"
SAR: "She must!"

October, 1985

"All the clinic patients I get are dumb, because all the smart ones switch to other doctors...."

March, 1987

JAR: "The patient is an 87-year-old priest who fainted while saying mass. The exact same thing happened 2 years ago, also while saying Mass."

SAR: "Has he only said Mass twice in 2 years?"
JAR: "Well, actually that's about the same as my attendance."

March, 1987

The intern, discussing a priest who has had two **syncopal** episodes while saying Mass: "This is what Joan of Arc had, and they didn't pace her. She'd talk to God, have a seizure, and that was it...they burned her at the stake."

July, 1988

The JAR, referring to a "sister" who had an **asystolic arrest**: "I guess you'd call her a 'blue nun'."

June, 1985

Regarding a patient with **IBD** who has long since overstayed her welcome for bowel arrest:
Intern: "The patient was wondering now what it takes to leave the hospital."
JAR: "I'll tell you what it takes. It takes my foot and her ass."

September, 1988

In regards to Mr. H:
JAR: "Neurologically, he's a jerk!"
SAR: (On the same patient): "**Foley** to traction!"

Quick retorts in the guise of doctors' orders often indicate anger. However, thoughts are different from actions, and these interventions were never actually ordered.

June, 1995

The SAR, to the **sleep apneic/Pickwickian** Mr. T, who was on a **Bigelow** team with him two years ago:
SAR: "Well, you don't look like you've lost any weight since I saw you last."
Mr. T: "Well, what can I say, neither have you!"

November, 1987

ICU patient, in for her 22nd admission, **status-post CABG**, to the team: "I'll give up smoking when you give up sex."
SAR: "So when do you give up smoking?"

December, 1998

Dr. S, on why she would not examine Mr. H's genitalia as part of his admission physical--"He's been in prison for ten years. I don't want to be the first woman in a decade to touch his penis--it just seems indecent. If he has any complaints of a **gonadal** nature, we can call Dr. L (A male resident)."

The boundaries between doctors and patients are not always rigid. Physicians can be chided by their patients and made publicly uncomfortable in the same way thoughtless physicians can shame their patients.

March, 1996

When our attending approached the 70-year-old woman with **primary pulmonary hypertension** without introduction, and **palpated** her right calf to assess for **DVT**--the mildly disgruntled patient was intact enough to react to this affront by slapping the attending on the back of his hand.

December, 1988

JAR: "I have a clinic patient coming in with what seems like a **GI** bleed. He's had 2 days of frank **melena** and is now dizzy."
SAR: "Any past medical history?"
JAR: "I follow him for **hypertension** and have been working him up for erectile dysfunction."
SAR: "Perhaps making him **hemodynamically stable** would help his potency..."

June, 1993

"It's like this--surgery would be loose stool, medicine would be formed stool for this guy's heart--it's shit either way."

January, 1995

Having a shitty morning. Moping around, feeling somewhat useless. Then, an uplifting event: Asked to talk to family regarding a husband, 44-year-old, **intubated** for severe pneumonia. You don't expect that telling a woman her husband is on the brink of death from **respiratory arrest** will be a pleasant experience. But, all of a sudden, for the first time while in the MICU, I gained a perspective, remembered why it is I'm doing this heinous, gruelling, torturous job. For the first time in the MICU, patients were real people, with real families, not some **gome** with a **TMax**, heart rate, **MAP**, **CVP**, **wedge**....

All of a sudden, in one sad 5-minute conversation, things made some sense and I felt pretty good.

May, 1993

SAR: "How was the patient's **mental status** during the procedure?"
Intern: "Oh fine. . . she was alert and completely with it; she yelled at me and threw me out of the room!"
SAR: "So, her judgment was intact . . ."

CHAPTER SIX

On Doctors

There are still times, maybe during a rare break from the hospital's chaos when I am sitting outside the MGH, just in front of the original Bulfinch building, that I cannot believe I have finished my residency. My journey began in seventh grade when, momentously (at least, momentous for me!), I moved my science folder in my Trapper Keeper in front of my English folder, thus declaring I would rather be a doctor than a journalist (my father's profession). In college I majored in biology, took the MCAT (Medical College Admission Test) – an eight-hour test. Quite a marathon!), and entered medical school in the Fall of 1991.

Most medical school programs are divided into two parts – the basic science curriculum during the first two years, which is mostly classroom-based with didactic lectures focusing on gross anatomy, biochemistry, physiology, pathology, and so on; and the clinical rotations curriculum, during which students work with different services in the hospital (internal medicine, surgery, pediatrics, obstetrics/gynecology, psychiatry) and in the office setting (primary care family practice, internal medicine, pediatrics, obstetrics/gynecology). Through these "apprenticeships," students start to learn how to care for patients and decide which field to enter. All medical students then enter a "match," which involves interviewing at a number of residency programs throughout the country and then ranking those programs in order of preference. At the same time, those programs rank the interviewing medical students in order of preference. Both sets of lists are entered into a computer, and at noon (derisively called: "High Noon!") on a designated day in the middle of March, each med student receives his or her match, the residency program he or she is assigned to attend, starting at the end of June or on July 1st.

Residency lasts anywhere from three to seven years, depending on the specialty. Afterwards, many residents enter a fellowship, in which they specialize within a field (for instance, a resident in an internal medicine residency may focus in cardiology). This additional training may last another one to five years. When you add up all the years of training, it is easy to see why some doctors do not "hang their shingle" until they are in their thirties! At this point, the doctor is considered an "attending" physician. At MGH, the attending is called a "visit." MGH, the third oldest hospital in the country, was established in the early 1800s to care for people who could not afford to have a doctor come to their home. The city of Boston also expected those "private" doctors to "visit" the hospital, to care for these people.

Residency is a continuation of the apprenticeship started in medical school. Internship, the first year of residency, can be a frightening and thrilling experience. Interns, the neophyte doctors, must learn an entirely new language – medspeak. They learn how to write orders, how to gather information from patients, family members, and from other hospitals, how to recognize patterns of illness, and how to distinguish among different diseases that can present the same way. For instance, a patient complaining of shortness of breath could have pneumonia, a heart attack, a blood clot to the lungs, a panic attack, or a toxic inhalation. Interns also learn how to order tests and how to perform procedures. The process of mastering all of the details that go into practicing medicine is often epitomized by the saying: "See one, do one, teach one." Second- and third-year residents continue this incredible learning experience, focusing more on recognizing different types of illness, managing disease, and teaching interns and medical students.

It is no wonder, then, that residency can be a stressful experience. When I trained, residents typically worked 70-120 hours per week (There are only 168 hours in a week – I've done the math!) and went

36-hour stretches without sleep (NB: Recently, duty hours across the nation have been capped at 80 hours per week). This lack of sleep colored everything and caused a wide spectrum of emotions to arise with a hair-trigger, ranging from giddiness to despondency to irritability. Despite sleep deprivation, residents must manage patients, "do" procedures (often after having only "seen" one performed), and respond to emergencies. Obviously, with all this time devoted to work, any semblance of an active social life dissolves; frequently families and relationships suffer, particularly during internship.

It is a wild ride. And it is truly heartening to see that your well-adjusted, well-rounded role models, your attendings, have left journal entries similar to yours when they were residents.

Mikkael Sekeres, M.D., M.S.

February, 1992

Dr. N tells us on rounds, "I used to be a dentist. My favorite movie was "Marathon Man.": You know the scene when the dentist tortures Dustin Hoffman?" Awkward silence follows.

June, 1998

Midnight Rounds--reading the charts.
Ortho Note: "Skin is taught about the right **iliac crest**."
  --What did the skin learn?

October, 1988

JAR: "The surgeon was here. I don't think they want to take the toe off. He wrote something about '**auto-amputation**.'"
Intern: "You mean they just want to let it fall off?"
JAR: "No, it means they want to have it run over by an auto."
Intern: "Can we write for that?"

July, 1997

Typical of our consults this month:
JAR (To **neurosurgeon**): "That **epidural collection** you **tapped** today has 2200 **white cells**. What does that mean?"
Neurosurgeon: "I don't know, so I'm going to ignore it."
JAR: "Assuming we care, what should we do about it?"
Neurosurgeon: "To be honest, we only tapped it because you kept bothering us; obviously that didn't work."

March, 1989

Dr. S (A psychiatrist) when asked if he thought that psychiatrists were ever vague in their answers: "Well, sometimes yes and sometimes no."

May, 1990

The attending, noting that the Pathology Department was extremely interested in a dying patient allegedly because of his **panhypoglobu-linemia**, states: "Did you see a pathologist up here rounding on Mr. I today? The guy's dying, but they're here doing like a **pre-cath**, but it's a pre--**post**. They dropped some orders on the chart. They're starting a **formaldehyde drip**."

Interdisciplinary squabbling runs rampant in hospitals. One group often refers to another as "they" and "they," in kind, criticize "us." Sayings and jokes that emphasize the popular stereotypes of specialties within medicine include:

Internists are doctors who know everything and do nothing.
Surgeons are doctors who know nothing and do everything.
Psychiatrists are doctors who know nothing and do nothing.
And pathologists are doctors who know everything and do every-thing, but too late.

An internist, psychiatrist, surgeon, and pathologist are in a boat to-gether while hunting. Suddenly, an object flies overhead.
The internist comments: "Well, that may be a bird, but our differential also has to include a cloud, a small plane, a pterodactyl, and a football."
The psychiatrist replies: "I wonder how the bird feels flying all alone like that."

The surgeon takes the gun and shoots the object, which falls into the water. He grabs it and hands it to the pathologist, demanding: "Tell me what it is."

December, 1987

An intern, after 1 month in the ICU: "Physical exam was remarkable for the **electroencephalogram** which showed..."

April, 1985

Attending to JAR: "You can stop the **prazosin**, or back off on the **paste**...or do whatever you want to do."
JAR to intern: "Do whatever you want to do."

As high technology becomes pervasive in ICUs, for some the physical examination has become a dying art. Physicians rely on objective data from machines, putting themselves at risk for missing the forest for the trees. When this happens, a sense of responsibility may be jeopardized.

May, 1992

Attending to JAR: "What would be an alternative explanation for this patient's pertinent findings, Dan?"
JAR: "I'm the wrong person to ask."
Attending: "Why?"
JAR: "Because I didn't hear the question."

August, 1991

During attending rounds discussing a patient's renal failure, the attending asks the intern: "Was the **creatinine** down to 2.7 or 2.3 today?"

The intern, fast asleep with her head in her hands, bolts up in her chair responding with confidence, "Yes!"

January, 1991

During attending rounds, the post-call intern had his head on the table and began loudly snoring. The JAR, finding him rather disruptive to rounds, was about to nudge him.
Attending: "Leave him alone—we've all been there."
JAR: "Yes...but not so loudly."
Our peal of laughter wakes up the blissful intern.

February, 1992

The JAR, after a disjointed, post-call interns' presentation: "She really needed to buy a vowel."

January, 1988

A 36-year-old man with **urinary retention** of 9 liters and **psychogenic polydipsia**:
SAR: "I can't believe that Mr. G. was able to keep 9 liters of urine in his bladder!"
JAR: "I know what you mean. I have a tough time just making it through rounds."

May, 1983

Just a note regarding what must be taken as a compliment by the administration on **Bigelow 8**: A screen was placed in front of our meeting room so our "discussions" would not be visualized.

Imagine being awake for 24 hours straight and feeling an urge to sleep that approaches pain. It is at that precise moment that rounds begin, often lasting five hours. Having just been on-call, these residents are the stars of the show; they present their night's work to a captive and often critical audience. Clarity of thought and enthusiasm give way to slumber during any instance of inactivity, or when attention is directed to another resident.

February, 1984

Quoting Dr. I: "What's the big deal, once you do a pelvic, you've done a pelvic! It's not like it's rocket science!!"

June, 1994

The intern's note of frustration while doing a speculum exam by accident on the rectum: "I can't see the cervix!"

Physicians often minimize the significance of tests and procedures that they order and perform on patients. This is done in part to keep their own anxiety in check, allowing them to perform in a competent, though not always confident, way.

April, 1998

HMS was intrigued with the preparation of a milk and molasses enema in room 9. But a concerned shadow soon spread over her face.
HMS: "After you give the enema, how do you know that what you're getting back is stool?"
Nurse: "Shit is shit."
I imagine truer words have never before been spoken.

<u>Addendum:</u> Later that night, the nurse emerges from room 9 with a concerned shadow on <u>her</u> face.
Nurse: "You know, that med student had a point . . . we put brown stuff in, we get brown stuff out!"

May, 1987

Discussing a **septic** patient:
Attending: "I assume you cultured him up the yazoo."
Intern: "We didn't **culture** his yazoo."

Patients with widespread infection have samples of blood, urine, stool, and spinal fluid taken in the hope of determining the location of the infection and the type of organism involved.

July, 1998

The SAR, speaking about disaster control, on what to do if Mr. B (**status-post** massive **GI** bleed) re-bleeds:
"First, blow up the **Blakemore**, get fluids going wide open, call GI, and then run around screaming, "Oh my God!" (Hands in air, eyes bugging out, etc.).

February, 1991

A male JAR and Dr. N were preparing to place a **central line** in a patient. The JAR was starting to put on his gown when a female resident coincidentally walked into the unit, spotted the JAR, and asked: "Do you want me to tie you up?"
Dr. N and I couldn't help but note the smirk behind the JAR's mask and a blush on the female resident's face.

A central line is a large catheter, or IV, placed into one of the veins in the neck or chest, allowing multiple IV medicines to be given at the same time, or a large volume of fluids (including blood or saline) to be administered quickly. The skin over the vein in which the catheter will be placed is cleaned with an antiseptic solution, betadine. Lidocaine, or Novacaine, is then injected just under the skin to numb-up the area. A small needle is inserted into the vein (called a "finder needle") to assure its location (these veins do not stick out like veins in the arm). A larger needle then is inserted into the vein based on the mapping of the finder needle, and a wire is threaded through the larger needle, into the vein. The larger needle is then removed with the physician still holding the end of the wire, the hole through which the wire enters the skin to the vein is enlarged with a scalpel, and a plastic dilator needle is advanced over the wire to enlarge the opening in the vein. This is then removed (with the wire still in place), and the final catheter is advanced over the wire into the vein. Finally, the wire is removed, and the catheter is sewn into place. This is known as the "Seldinger" technique.

June, 1998

With reference to a patient's spiking fever to 105°:
SAR: "If we could only harness that heat. . ."

June, 1982

"It's hard to improve upon a patient who is not sick to begin with."

August, 1985

Dr. G, in reference to the ICU team: "I don't own this gas station, I just pump the gas."

ON DOCTORS

October, 1987

The intern, referring to a patient who had not improved in spite of vigorous efforts of the ICU team: "We've been **buffing** him for a week... but he ain't shining!"

March, 1985

Dr. B (A cardiologist): "We have definitely established that the heart is putting out the calls, but the kidneys aren't picking up the phone."

September, 1981

Late at night when no one is around except the memories inscribed, we allow the stored up and unprocessed feelings to flood onto this paper. It is very helpful—but how sad it is that it is so rare that we share the feelings with ourselves and with each other. Hour after hour, the visceral sensations give us clues that something is wrong, or right, within us. Nausea, **tachycardia**, cramping—how much easier I feel these and enjoy sadness or despair. A respirator is turned off, a patient's heart stops, a family grieves. This, I say, must be an important landmark in my life—I am experiencing the care of existence—so many of the emotions and substance of being are encompassed by this experience—but before I can process any of this experience, I must move on. I hope to go home and to think and to feel and to write about the experience—but at home I want to put the hospital completely behind me—and so it goes—until we sit with this book in front of us and finally process some of these visceral sensations.

May, 1984

Sometimes you have to steal away to gain your control or you lock the bathroom door and cry. I'd almost never cried before I became

139

an intern. I used to dread my mornings on—when I'd face the judgment of the team the morning after—because I'd "**crump**" when they looked over my orders or listened to what I'd done and either talked about alternative plans or criticized those I'd opted for. I nearly always had an awful catch in the throat and three times split at the earliest possible moment to bawl like a child in some bathroom somewhere.... and sure, there's anger beneath it all that you cannot express and don't wish to acknowledge. Anger over the fact that others don't appreciate you when what you really want is to be loved and valued, anger that people badger you to do things, and the more you do the less you're thanked. Anger when someone tells you that you're incredibly slow in presenting patients and then seeing the same person deliver the most conspicuously slow and halting summary of a patient's presenting problems and further care. Angry at the petty digs by others, the minor and major cruelties. I keep on marveling at how nice the people here are—they're fantastic—but some of the deliberate cruelties practiced here are amazing. I can't bear to be more specific. There are great moments—you're on top of the world—when you've been congratulated for a fine job, when you've helped a family through a tough time or cleared the confusion, when you see the chance to really help a house officer or nurse or whoever through a bind. It is the unpredictability that is so problematic. We're emotional time bombs, terrible cliché that it is. Nothing is more vexatious.

June, 1985

I've never felt so incompetent as I felt today.

November 25, 1986

The day before Thanksgiving. Why is it that it gets harder and harder to put things in perspective? My favorite time of day is post-call, when I can hide my white jacket, stethoscope, and beeper and slip into the crowds of visitors unnoticed. The world swimming hazily before my eyes. Then perhaps I'll sit for awhile over my onion rings or microwave bagel, a comfortable distance away from other solitary lunchers. It seems that such times are the only times my life intersects with reality. For the rest, I am playing a role, a name I don't answer to naturally. The only honest ones are those who tell me right out that I'm not ready to be a doctor.

January, 1982

Do I try to remember my feelings to bring them back to life so that others can see them: "I'm the only one who feels this way—I'm the only one who doesn't understand what's going on—I'm scared, angry, tired, sad, incompetent, weak, pressured, lonely, isolated, bitter, dumb, inefficient, and nobody else could feel as I do."

IT'S NOT TRUE!--We all feel that. We all look for the crack of dawn that signals the passage of responsibility to a fresh crew. We all know the system sucks, that the long hours make for fuzzy thinking and that they generate pure blind hate at facing that next ridiculous admission. We all feel the frustration of doing too much for too few, and the insecurity of not knowing how much is too much or if it was really too little. We don't like admitting how little we know, and none of us wants to look like fools. We don't like criticism and yet we need it. We **flog** and flog, and rarely have the opportunity to see the veritable forest for the trees. We hate the patients for making more work for us. We especially hate the grossly self-destructive ones who don't deserve our sweat and society's money.

And yet we get some satisfaction from some things. We derive lots of personal pride in procedures well done, in a code well run, in a diagnosis astutely made, regardless if the patient lives or dies. We derive satisfaction from the few sick patients with reversible illness who live and live well as a result of our interventions. And, although it's too little in coming, we derive a lot, perhaps the most, satisfaction and pride in getting positive feedback from our peers and immediate superiors. Remember that! Don't be jealous. Your time will come. Give that pat on the back, and give it with heartfelt genuineness. You'll know that, coming from those who work as you do, the compliment will mean more than those from the patients or even the nurses. There are those who you can fool, and those you can't. A whiff of esprit de corps is overpowering.

For many individuals who have become physicians, the goal of being emotionally available and sensitive to their patients seems lost during the years as a houseofficer. Listening may become a chore which results in one feeling overwhelmed. Ironically, in attempting to maintain compassion towards their patients during extremely physically and emotionally challenging years, houseofficers become insensitive to each others' needs.

October, 1994

When I'm on call, my fish are on call, they eat and sleep when I get home, however, they never complain.

March, 1993

JAR: "The patient was alert and oriented, but would slip into a slumberous state without constant stimulation."

The attending grins and points to the sleeping intern who, upon being poked, wakes up momentarily, smiles, and then drifts into sleep once again as the JAR continues her presentation.

February, 1991

"I would sleep all the time if gluttony did not overcome sloth."

--Dr. A, who loves scarfing coffee and doughnuts on morning rounds.

June 24, 1994

So here it is the last night of internship in the Bigelow unit and the last page of this volume of the house staff journal. What a year. I didn't quite learn a bunch of things that I thought I would...it seems like just yesterday I was taking notes on how to write **Colace** orders (now is that **p.o.** or **p.r.**) but it's 4 a.m. and I think I'm beginning to hallucinate—the **I-meds** sound a little bit like crickets...I gaze out the window at the immense darkness, and I think to myself, "How insignificant you are, you meager little peon." But then again, I thought that yesterday, too, and I wasn't even near a window.

I will dearly miss all these people here...all these people are my family now, and to all of them in these last wee hours of internship, I take great pride in saying: "I just want all of you to know how much I respect you and have enjoyed working with you." Bye.

June 24, 1985

So this is it.
The clock strikes midnight on my last night in the
Intensive care unit and
My last day of senior residency.
The beeper is turned to off.

I am standing on the roof of the apartment, the warm
Spring night before this all began, or walking home on a
Cold New Year's Day morning after a long night on call
In the **Phillips House**.
Or escaping for one day in the bright fall to pick apples.

I am bleary eyed, standing in the stairwell at 2 a.m., shaking
Or laughing my guts out, post call.

I am sleeping in a summer breeze, I am falling in love.

I am watching the street person going through the garbage in
The dark, looking for something to eat. When was the time that a
Sight like this would bring tears to my eyes?

Residency is mainly a test of bravery.
Our courage grows in these three years.
We try our best, our knowledge is imperfect, but
We work under the guise of perfection.
Confidence reduced to mere style.

We understand some things about each other.
It is one thing being up together and working with you so closely
All through the night.
There is nothing that compares with seeing your smiling faces
In the morning.

To fearlessness without callousness.
Love to all my dear friends on the house staff....

*It often takes the stimulus of emotional lability encountered early in
the morning after a grueling month's long rotation for the softer under-
belly of emotion to ooze out. Sentimentality may not seem deep or heartfelt; but that superficiality itself may be a cover.*

January, 1999

In desperation at the filthiness of the JAR's white coat, the intern
took the coat, after the JAR had left post-call, down to the Facilities
Management Office, to trade it in for a new one. After much arguing
and cajoling, the intern was able to obtain a new coat.
The Group: "So, you got a new coat yesterday?"

JAR: "Yeah, but they said the old coat was so dirty that they just threw it out!"
SAR: "You mean they withdrew on your coat?"
JAR: Yeah, I think they counted it as an ethical save."

June, 1997

Intern: "Why do they call it '**Optimum Care**?'
SAR: "Because if they called it 'really sucky advice from ethicists,' no one would consult them."

The humorous punch-line at the end of some of these entries is meant to mask anger.

January, 1983

The **cardiothoracic** surgeon, after telling a patient **status-post MI** and **CABG** with an **occluded graft**, that he had a 30% chance of dying the next day: "You're a damned fool to keep smoking, you're wasting my talents." Harsh.

November, 1992

JAR, on a patient who was a Benedictine monk, and who refused a **central line**: "He may be close to God with what he does, but so are we!"

September, 1990

Says the consulting **neurologist**, regarding: the deplorable consult he gets.
"My favorite? A consult for 'mental stroke.' Diagnosis: Stroke of genius."

May, 1997

FYBIGMI at its best (Fuck you Buddy, I've got my internship):
HMS (Illinois-bound in Orthopedics) with hands behind head and leaning back in his chair, unwisely only doing one night of call this week: "I've already done enough call."

What makes people arrogant? No doubt, many causes. For some, arrogance is a defense against personal feelings of inadequacy, a condition that most arrogant individuals would reject. But when doctors behave in an arrogant fashion, it usually detracts from the care of patients.

June, 1992

The SAR, in the midst of a raging discussion about the answer to tomorrow's trivia contest question: "I used to know baseball trivia. Then I had to replace it with medical minutia."

November 30, 1991

The attending, when pondering a patient with poor **ABGs** and a question of poor **central drive**, commented that "her low **PO2** probably is worsened when she is asleep. Remember that for the respiratory system, sleep is a stress."
Dr. A: "If that's so, stress me more."

May, 1990

On discussing inappropriate pages: one resident: "I was called at 4 a.m. by an operator who said, 'I just wanted to check on how I could reach you!'"

146

December, 1987

JAR: "I mean the worst thing about residency is that you can't keep up with what's going on in the real world—I didn't know Black Monday had occurred until Tuesday!"

May, 1991

At sign-out rounds Dr. L asked several questions about Mrs. O's **septic P-A line** numbers. The SAR, referring to a recent paper, asks: "L, do you get the **Annals**?"
Dr. L replies: "The Annals? I don't even get the Boston Globe!"

August, 1994

Commenting on movies watched by a patient last night--"Rear Window," "City Slickers," Dr. U laments, "She has a better social life than all of us combined!"

March, 1993

Dr. X, in discussing an irritable prisoner who took an antidepressant overdose to evade arrest, "How about if I go to jail and she stays to be on call?"

A physician's vulnerabilities often are unearthed by a variety of stressors: endless information that must be incorporated; sleep deprivation; and a disconnect from the realities of the non-medical world. Particularly in the MICU, where residents are even isolated from the rest of their colleagues, the notion of the "hospital as a prison" takes on an even greater reality.

October, 1989

Older physicians claim that we will all eventually look back on our internships with fondness. I find that a little bit hard to believe right now, but who knows what a little dementia might bring.

April, 1991

Sign-out rounds.
SAR to **HMS**: "What are the mechanisms of **VT**?"
HMS: "That's definitely a junior-level question."
SAR: "And that's not a medical student-level comment!"

February 28, 1996

"I hate Leap Year!" On being on call February 29th."

February, 1983

Well, I'm back as the resident, and the intern is writing those G-D unit notes, and the only reason I'm not in the sack is that it's 7:30 p.m. and who wants to have the operator give you a wake-up call for the evening meal...the anger, fear, and frustration that marked my earlier entries in this book have been diffused somewhat by virtue of the great pacifier—sleep. It's incredible what a few hours of undisturbed slumber can make. I can smile lugubriously at the total body failures that call us at 3 a.m. because I don't have be up till 7 a.m. writing them up—rage is an intern's emotion. At times, I miss the deliciously self-righteous rage that only an exhausted intern can feel—but I would not trade my sleep for that emotion.

June, 1993

What if we indeed won and vanquished death, so that only a memory remains? I would live forever and ever. . . I would be **Osler** in 200 years, cluttering the medical world with meaningless thoughts and words. Would I be happy sharing my world with 58 trillion other people around? People everywhere, just keep on coming. . . making love without castration would have to be outlawed. . . just to make room for all the old fogies that now have immortality. What a nightmare . . . In a sense, ICUs are a small price to pay for the ever-present certainty of cleansing, releasing, regenerating death.

October, 1993

"We don't really know anything. The more I see, the more I'm convinced of that. We just do our rituals--we have our consultants and pat each other on the backs.

May, 1996

"If you're going to do nothing, you might as well do it at high doses."

February, 1993

We've run out of things to do for her, and now, we're just doing things to her.

Sometimes it is possible to lose sight of the big picture. Critically ill individuals often lose the possibility of a meaningful life as their ability to communicate and function ebbs. Faced with this day-by-day slippage of humanity, house officers may revert to unilateral decisions, oversimplified realities, cynicism, and cries of futility.

June, 1992

JAR: "Mr. H is going to leave us today."
SAR: "Mr. H has already left us. We're just going to stop bothering him."

October, 1986

On rounds:
JAR: "Well actually the only reason why we decided to keep this **soft rule-out** patient is that he can be enrolled in the **MI** study, and that means pizza money."
Attending: "Seems like house officers would do anything for money."
JAR: "That's why they call us **H.O.**'s."

Some research studies offered "prizes," or finders' fees, to doctors who recruit patients to those studies.

June, 1995

It's been 2 years since orientation. Two years since our first get-together lunch, when I met the green interns before the games began. Two years since a rising star M.D./Ph.D. colleague pulled me aside and said: "I'm not sure I'm supposed to be here." Who was at the time?

It's funny, but looking back, I find it hard to remember the bad times. After seeing first-hand and sharing in (the best proper word) the most personal and painful feelings any human being can take, who could have the gall to complain? When you've seen a couple of nice patients with AIDS--most of life's problems seem dwarfed. Am I the only one who thinks this disease is fucking bizarre?! We've sequenced the entire HIV **genome** and can make it jump molecular hoops in a test-tube, but still, they die like skeletons. And most of them seem to be my age! Okay, so perhaps I'm venting, but they're with me. I'm sure when I get older and have the first twinge of

squirrelly chest pain, I'll have the same angst towards coronary artery disease.

When I look at what I find on a daily basis, I'm surprised that I had the will to wake up in the morning. Tonight, for instance, we performed the flog-the-old-demented-man-with-painful-procedures-until-his-wife-signs-the-DNR-orders routine to perfection. We've turned up the **FIO$_2$**, down the **peep**, up the insulin, pulled the **A-line**, got the consent, pleased the nurses, gave the Haldol, did the CT transport, wrote the orders, ordered the take-out food, watched "Nightline," ran the books, changed the antibiotics, talked to the Medford Police, drew the blood cultures, and walked the halls in search of late night gossip.

When I look at what I've learned over the last two years, I'm humbled by the outcomes of our rather crude medical technology. That some of this shit works amazes me, but most of it doesn't make sense. In 20 years, fellow interns will look back and think we were all in the stone age--like a bunch of medical cavemen, groping for the medicinal fire. At least, I hope they will. Here's to the evolution.

June, 1986

Our **visit**: "I try hard not to be <u>just</u> a doctor."

March, 1980

The smart man knows that simple things are important. The very smart man knows that simple things are very important. The brilliant man knows that simple things are very important but not all important things are simple.

November, 1986

Assumption is the mother of fuck-up.

January, 1981

As I read all the really profound notes in this journal, I realize that basically, this lifestyle just ain't fucking normal.

One of our colleagues said: "Lack of an adequate response (to a crack, an insult) results in gibberish or violence. In this case, the residents use cursing (violence) to respond to untenable situations.

July, 1986

Dr. P (JAR) to intern after the first week of internship on the ICU team: "Let's go in and see the patient. Then you can decide how much **lasix** I want to give him."

September, 1998

The attending gave a lunchtime talk today, and shattered what little confidence I had in my grasp of **MAP**'s, **CVP**'s, **tissue perfusion pressures**, and so on.

For whatever reason, it reminded me of the story of a man walking in the park, who stumbled across a second man, down on all fours, combing the grass under a street lamp for something lost. The first man asked the 2nd what he's lost. "My keys," man #2 says.
"Whereabouts did you lose them?" Man #1 says.
"Over there," says man #2, pointing him to the dark, dense bushes 20 yards away.
"But why are you looking here?" Asked man #1.
Man #2 says: "This is where the light is."

April, 1980

The last night on the Bigelow ICU. The last night on the Bigelow, period. Let me restate, first things first. About internship: nothing in house staff training compares with the intensity and impact of sudden terrific (as in Melville, terror-ific) awareness of the palpable absurdity in what we so often actually do as when it comes through the numbing film of months of chronic sleep deprivation. It seems in retrospect something like big strobe lights suddenly only feet away, enjoy. And nothing compares with the pain of pushing back sleep again and again. You may some day miss the former but never the latter.

April, 1980

Not all accounts in this book will be as vivid or packed with emotion as was the last entry—but that doesn't make it less important for us.

A lesson to be learned is that all of us have had those feelings—and it is essential to remember that feelings are different from actions—the consequences of them make them different.

The hazard we face is forgetting what it's like being up all night; having all the responsibility; while feeling little appreciated.

The more we are able to use our memories, the easier it will be to take care of people in the future. Keep up the good work and keep pen to paper.

T Stern

June, 1996

Optimum Care Committee: The committee has decided that it is in the best interest of intern T, the house staff, and the ICU patients, that T be provided safe passage off the MICU Service. The efforts of the doctors to instruct him in the mores and knowledge base of a clinician are recognized and appreciated, but to continue to attempt to force knowledge into a person as dull and thick-skulled as T, would be viewed as nothing more than cruel and inhuman torture. If any further help is needed in escorting Dr. T, who has devoted his life to maintaining his blissful ignorance of internal medicine, off the service, please contact me.

P.S. Thanks for the teaching these last two weeks. I've enjoyed it very much.

Signed: Dr. T

June 24, 1986—3 a.m.

After 12 months of trial by fire, I'm ready for some more responsibility and I'm excited about the opportunity to share some of my newfound knowledge with the next group of terrified MGH house officers. Good luck to you all—and thanks everybody.

June 30, 1992

Dr. M: "You should write something profound about the first few days." I'm tired.

June, 1981

S:
Not so long ago
I used to get
Distracted
By the faces of ICU patients. So,
Filled
With emotion, bursting with pain and dread,
Lying half-naked, half-dead
Among the tubes and machines
That suck and blow.

O:
No time for that now. More
Important
Matters to attend to:
Unit notes, beepers, and such.

A:
I am learning.
Now, I see no faces behind the oxygen masks,
Only **wedge pressure** tracings,
Urine outputs,
And **EKG**'s.
It's all I have time for.

P:
At last,
I am becoming a doctor.

June, 1985

Now leaving my ICU time as the SAR, I'm less inclined to be bitter and to criticize many of our ridiculous habits and rules...and more inclined to be "seniorly" and to give out "fatherly" advice to the new interns and interns to be. Several points I've come to appreciate:

1. I still hurt when someone dies and I still feel very helpless at times despite knowing a few more tricks.
2. To be 100% M.D. and 0% human is a shallow existence. Get out of the fucking hospital every now and then and enjoy life.
3. Be cautious of others' opinions—remember...opinions are like assholes—everybody's got one and everybody else's stinks!

4. Enjoy your time here because as it seems long now at the end it is short. Despite its shortcomings you will look back with pride and fondness (I wouldn't really want to repeat though!).

5. "Gallows humor" is okay. You need the release. Don't be afraid to let it out (in private).

6. Lastly my secret of survival—my favorite quote (author unknown to me): There are three kinds of time: goal achieving, tension relieving, and a waste of time. Maximize the first two and eliminate the last and you will be successful and happy.

June 24, 1994

10:00 p.m., last day of MICU, last day of internship. Finally finished off last service note. Now officially done with internship. Need something profound to say. . . Oh, fuck. . . It's 10 p.m.. . .I'm not on call. . . I eat dinner here. . . I'm a loser. . . Good luck new interns.

Post-script:
Surviving the ICU

We had three "family meetings" in the last 24 hours. A family meeting has a special meaning in the ICU; most of the time it is convened to deliver bad news. Rarely is everyone called together to provide news of dramatic improvement. Who needs to? We do that at the bedside, in the waiting room, and in the hallway. We even yell it at the patient: "You are getting better!!," who most often forgets what we said anyway.

The goal of many family meetings is to communicate to a distraught family that we think there is little hope of cure or survival for a loved one, i.e., nothing we can do will work. Since their loved one is not getting better with the treatment we're providing, we should start thinking about "withdrawing support," "capping therapy," and not resuscitating that person should a catastrophic event occur, i.e., make him or her Do Not Resuscitate (DNR), and "make her comfortable." Typically having these discussions means that *we* did not succeed; i.e., we exhausted our resources, the heights to which technology has taken us, and have run out of further technology, medicine, and ideas to manage critical illness.

Being at a family meeting is one of the most intense emotional experiences one can have while working in an ICU. However, while stressful, it can also result in an emotional high as well. Most of the time we stop using medical jargon and the language of the trade (e.g., by explaining ambiguous values and measurements), and we use the straight-talking language of the family, who is often scared-to-death. It is the time we most connect with people. It is often a time to let go; we are different after leaving a family meeting.

At these meetings, I have met all sorts of people. White, Black, Irish, Italian, Indian, and Oriental. Rich, poor, and middle class. English speaking, as well as Portugese, Cambodian, and others. When Italian is required I feel quite comfortable. Some family members sit silently, some scream, and a few are very angry; all of them are sad, they hug each other, and they cry. Frequently, I leave the room after a family meeting with a knot in my throat. Meetings are often joined by a priest, pastor, minister, rabbi, imam, or a Buddhist monk. I had not known what an imam was until we had to talk with a very religious Moroccan family. I had never seen a Buddhist monk before one such meeting. I prayed with all of them, despite the fact that on many occasions I did not know what they were saying; it didn't really matter. Ironically, it was at these moments, that I felt that I could be really helpful. *"We all must die. But that I can save him from days of torture, that is what I feel as my ever new privilege. Pain is an even more terrible lord of mankind than death itself"*. (Dr. Albert Schweitzer, 1931).

At times family meetings can be less than friendly. Family members who have been hurt by terrible tragedy may develop doubts about the adequacy of our care. This tension can be hard to bear. For example, take Mr. A, a man in his forties. Two months earlier he had surgery for a perforated stomach ulcer that was complicated by a "leak" from one of his sutures. Repeated infections developed in his abdomen, which were very difficult to control. He was transferred to our Surgical ICU, unconscious, and on a ventilator. Despite receiving the most powerful antibiotics, numerous medications to perfuse his damaged and exhausted organs, he was still critically ill. Because he was receiving extraordinary amounts of sedatives and narcotics to maintain his comfort it was impossible to tell whether his brain was still functional. Four months into this devastating illness, some of us started to wonder: "How much longer can, and should, this go on?" Clinical experience and scientific data suggest that, on the average, the chance that a critically ill patient will die increases with the length of stay in the ICU and with the number of vital organ systems (e.g., the lungs, the kidneys, and the brain) that require artificial support. Had any of these means of support been discontinued, he would have died quickly. The chance of him surviving his ICU stay was far less than 10%.

We told the family about our concerns. He lived with his mother, who at first I thought was not very inquisitive; she came to visit him only infrequently, yet she called to see how he was doing every night. Later, I realized that she just could not bear to see her son in the ICU. Mr. A had a very outspoken brother and sister-in-law; they asked specific medical questions and they kept notes about our answers. The healthcare team was not unanimous about his dismal prognosis. He did not have a terminal disease, he had not destroyed any of his vital organs and, probably most important, he was young. The atmosphere in our meeting with his family was unusually tense. His brother and sister-in-law greeted me while holding a tape recorder: "Do you mind if we record what you say?" They confronted me with specific questions already written on a legal pad and they compared my responses with those of other doctors that they previously interviewed. His mother just listened; it did not take much to convince her to give us more time.

After a couple more weeks, Mr. A started to get better. Four weeks later, we transferred him to our Respiratory Unit to complete his wean from the ventilator. It was clear that Mr. A would survive. His mother started coming in daily and she sat at his bedside for longer and longer periods. Two months after he left our Respiratory Unit, and more than half a year into his illness, she sent us a photograph of him; he was off the ventilator, standing up, and smiling. It was addressed "to her Angels in the ICU." While I don't think we are angels, I believe that Mr. A had someone special looking down on him.

Sometimes caregivers disagree with each other. ICU patients are extremely complicated, both medically and ethically. For some of us, it is easier to continue to push medical care beyond heroic efforts than to confront the inevitability of failure.

Mr. B, a young man whom I cared for a few years ago in our SICU, came to us after an enormous operation; his surgeon had tried to eliminate a cancerous growth from the hip bone. His cancer had spread to other vital organs, and his only hope, chemotherapy, was not considered to be a viable option. He deteriorated rapidly after the massive surgery. He required high doses of medications to maintain an adequate blood pressure and his kidneys started to fail. Everyone (except his surgeon) in the ICU knew Mr. B was going to die. At a late night family meeting, the surgeon declared "We are not going to give up!;" he then turned to me and said, "If he was your father, you wouldn't give up either!". The surgeon had not known that I had already been through this a long time ago with my own father and mother; I was way ahead of him. Mr. B expired three days later. As is the case when any young person dies, it was very distressing. In addition to our sense of loss, our obvious disagreement left us with a bitter taste. This tainted my relationship with him; I had liked the surgeon, a fatherly figure. He was kind to everybody, and interactions with him always left others with a favorable impression.

About two years later, the same surgeon, by then retired, stopped me in the hallway and said, "Luca, I just came back from burying my sister. She died of cancer. She was in an ICU for a long time and we decided to withdraw support. She died peacefully." We shook hands, for the first time in two years. Now he stops and picks me up at the corner of Beacon Street where I wait for public transportation in the morning. Although he is retired he can't stay away from the hospital; he arrives at six-thirty in the morning. I admire this old man; despite his academic clout and incredible professional success, he was able to change his mind.

Not infrequently, there is no time for a family meeting, and the end arrives quickly. We move between rooms, make phone calls, and perform procedures. A life ends and it's over, but only for us, and really, not even for us.

On a chilly Saturday morning, rounds were disrupted by the arrival of Mr. C, a young construction worker who had fallen from a height of 30 feet. It had taken 45 minutes to extricate him from debris; he was found pulseless, unconscious, and cold. He had sustained a horrible blow to his head and had come to us with little more than a heart beat. As we abandoned our rounds and started working on his *other* problems, such as a low body temperature and an irregular heartbeat, it became clear that his mind was gone, blood was not perfusing his brain. His family looked frightened; they trickled in as they received the news of the accident. His father was a quiet man of about my age, who was trying to focus on the events and to plan accordingly; he was accustomed to making decisions, but he was barely able to speak. Shyly he asked me, if he could consult a friend of his, a neurosurgeon from another hospital. I brought him to my office and left him alone to make phone calls. Things continued to deteriorate and it was clear that Mr. C was going to die quite soon. I met with his mother, his devastated wife, and others, although I wasn't sure who they were. His dad left a message for the neurosurgeon. We discussed the possibility of organ donation, others were more focused on how the accident could have occurred. They knew that he had too much to drink the night before, but he had slept it off at a friend's place before he returned home. A lot of us were crying, too. By the time I left, all of the plans were made, and the family was more at peace with his passing. His dad hugged and thanked me.

Soon thereafter, I left to spend a year-long sabbatical in Italy. On my first Saturday back, a man in the waiting room asked to see me. He looked vaguely familiar, and was about my age. He smiled and greeted me: "They told me you were back. How was Italy?" As I finally recognized him, from that chilly spring morning a year earlier, I was stunned. He was Mr. C's father. He just wanted to say hello to some of the people he had met following his son's accident, an event that had changed his life forever.

Sometimes against all odds, things go well. Ms. D, a young woman who nearly drowned, required intensive care. Near-drowning may result in acute respiratory distress syndrome (ARDS), a form of respiratory failure about which we know little, except that it kills the majority of those who develop it. Nearly drowning fills the lungs with water; damage results from what's in the water. During my sabbatical I fine-tuned my knowledge and experience of the treatment of acute respiratory failure; hence, one of my colleagues asked me to consult on Ms. D. Ms. D's mother was there; she spoke very little and when she did it was only in Spanish. She never left the bedside. Ms. D was desperately ill. Every change in her ventilator settings I attempted further worsened her condition. I left a little disappointed, both for Ms. D and for my own pride. My colleagues suggested that we try extracorporeal membrane oxygenation (ECMO), a highly sophisticated technology where blood is circulated outside the body through an "oxygenator," a machine that essentially substitutes for the lungs on a temporary basis, while one hopes the lungs will start to heal. Despite my objections, she was placed on ECMO, and she remained near death for another week or so. I thought she was going to die. Two weeks later, Ms. D started to improve. Her mother even said a few words and at times went home. Ms. D came off ECMO, and continued to get better.

One night the following year, I went with my son to the Boston Garden to watch a basketball game between the Celtics and the Sixers. These games are no longer just about watching basketball. There is always something else occurring on the court: they throw t-shirts at the public, present all sorts of games and charities, and introduce amazing people. As the Sixers star, Alan Iverson was destroying the Celtics (while I was still dreaming that Bird, McHale, and Parish would walk onto the parquet floor) they introduced a young person that had done something exceptional. This woman was receiving the award for her courage facing a long illness; she had nearly drowned and doctors at the MGH had put her on a "heart-lung machine"..... *Ms. D!* She ran onto the court, smiling to everyone, and clapping her hands in joy. "I know her!" I told my son, Antonio, and I felt a little awkward. Although I had not been responsible for her care, I had tried to help; I had not done any good. Thank God somebody did. This is the beauty of a great hospital: there is always someone else who can help. ECMO worked, a young life was saved, I rejoiced with the crowd!

You always carry with you doubts about your abilities, no matter what stage of training you've entered. One night during my residency, one of my fellow residents covering another ICU called for help: a patient of one of the service's senior thoracic surgeons had "lost his airway." This was a rare but frightening nightmare in the ICU. Managing this surgeon's patients was problematic because their delicate tracheal reconstructions left the anatomy of the airway altered; should they decompensate ("loose their airway") it may be extremely difficult to find the airway. We needed to re-establish the patient's airway and help him breathe; if we were unable to do so he would die. I gave it my best shot, and placed the tube where I thought it should go; this enabled us to send him back to the Operating Room for a more definitive repair. Frightened and shaken by the thought that I had erred I returned to my ICU and got ready for morning report. I was devastated. I could not stop thinking about the patient. I did not even know his name. I felt that I had probably placed the tube in the wrong place, and disrupted the fine surgical work that only one surgeon in the world could have done. I thought of a fellow Intern in my residency program who would always say "They are going to throw me out of the Program!" I became convinced they would throw me out of the Program, even though I was not in their Program. I survived morning report, went home, and retreated to my bed. When I awoke, I found a message that my wife, Pat, left for me before going to work: "Dr. W from the MGH called. He said that the tube was in the right place. Thought you were very worried and that you would want to know. He said, "Good job."

Sometimes our most severely ill patients survive. Obviously it's more than sometimes, but we forget quickly about our successes. One after another patients come in; each requires our attention, each has his or her own story and family, and each generates new discussions and intense emotions. We tend to forget about those who have left the ICU; however, sometimes they return. It may be a few weeks to months later, when they finally are discharged from the rehabilitation hospital. Sometimes they stop by on their way to or from a follow-up visit with their surgeon. He or she sends them to us, to share with us the joy of seeing what the person looks like when they can once again walk and talk. We often have a hard time recognizing them: a beautiful young girl, a dignified elderly gentleman, a mother, a son, or a boyfriend: it was often hard to see them as having these roles when they are in the ICU. Often I recognize them from their pictures. ICU nurses learned long ago the benefits of thinking of patients as regular people. So, they ask family members to bring in pictures of the patient; and pretty soon the room is covered with photos of smiling people, kids, grandparents, and pets. Sometimes it is hard to tell which one in the photograph is the patient. Often, while we make rounds, I stop and stare at the pictures: "So, this is what she really looks like!"

Mrs. E, an 83-year-old woman, fell from her first floor balcony and sustained a series of injuries, the most important of which was a crush injury of her right chest as well as a neck fracture. Her fracture was what physicians call a "hangman fracture" (i.e., the cervical spine fracture sustained in a hanging): fortunately, she was lucky and she did not injure her spinal cord. She needed tubes in her chest to deal with internal bleeding and a hard collar around her neck to immobilize the fracture. She required a tracheostomy and a respirator to enable her breathe; eventually, she was transferred to our Respiratory Unit to complete the "weaning" from the respirator. However, it became clear that she had not taken care of herself: her lungs bore the signs of her having been a heavy smoker; in addition, she had not taken medications for high blood pressure. Her home situation was not much better. Her husband had been terminally ill when the accident occurred. We started to wonder about the fall, and whether it had been just an accident. The moment she could express herself clearly, she stated that she wanted to die and did not want further treatment. Long discussions with the family ensued and a psychiatric consultant diagnosed her as being depressed; we did not honor her request (because she lacked the capacity to make medical decisions while depression colored her judgment) and we pressed on. Her family was very asser-tive, of tough New England stock; they decided she was going to live. I had trouble dealing with that. I felt for her, particularly as she lost her husband. She had not been interested in medical care before her injury and she was even less interested in it now. Slowly she improved and she was transferred to the rehabilitation hospital.

One afternoon about four weeks later, Mrs. E's daughter strolled in, pushing a wheelchair. In the chair was an incredibly thin but smil-ing woman. Mrs. E was back; she was breathing, talking, and collect-ing the applause, the hugs, the jaw- dropping comments, and a few tears. Her daughter was beaming. When another physician in our group saw Mrs. E he asked her out, and everyone laughed. I felt a little ashamed for having thought that she wasn't going to make it. Then I said, "What the heck" and I joined in the celebration.

Luca Bigatello, M.D., Director of Surgical Critical Care,
St. Elizabeth Hospital, Salem, Massachusetts.

GLOSSARY OF TERMS

A

ABG: Arterial Blood Gas, a blood test measuring how well a person is getting oxygen into the blood

ABG Tube: Arterial Blood Gas, a blood test measuring how well a person is getting oxygen into the blood.

Acid-Base Disorders: Diseases that affect the relative acidity of the blood

Acidotic: A condition involving reduced alkalinity of the blood

ACLS: Advanced Cardiac Life Support, CPR with use of cardiac paddles, medications, and intubation

Acute: Of recent onset

Agonal: A pattern of breathing prior to death

AKA: Above the Knee Amputation

A-Line: Arterial line, an arterial catheter for blood pressure monitoring

Allen Street: The MGH morgue

Allen Street Table: The stretcher used to transport a corpse to the morgue

AMA: To leave the hospital Against Medical Advice

Ambu Bag: Ambulatory Bag, for use in "bagging"

Amps: Ampules, a pre-measured amount of medication.

Amnestic: Causing amnesia

Angiocaths: Intravenous catheters or needles

Annals: Short for the *Annals of Internal Medicine*, a medical journal

Anoxic: Insufficient oxygen

Anoxic Brain Damage: Insufficient oxygen to the brain causing injury

Anoxic Encephalopathy: Brain damage from insufficient oxygen supply

Anterolateral: The front and side of the heart

Anxiolytic: A medication treating anxiety
Aortic Dissection: A tearing of the wall of the aorta
Aortic Graft: A material placed to repair the wall of the aorta
Aortic Insufficiency: A malfunctioning type of heart valve
Aortic Stenosis: An abnormality of a heart valve
Aortic Valve: A heart valve
Aphasic: Unable to speak
Apneic: Not breathing
ARDS: Adult Respiratory Distress Syndrome, a severe lung disease that can be end-stage
Arrest: Cardiac Arrest, a state when the heart stops pumping blood
Arrhythmia: An abnormal heart rhythm
Arterial line: An arterial catheter for blood pressure monitoring
Art-line: Short for Arterial Line, an arterial catheter for blood pressure monitoring
AS: Aortic Stenosis, an abnormality of a heart valve
Aspirate: When food mistakenly goes down the trachea or wind pipe
Asthmatic: Suffering from severe asthma, unable to breathe
Asystole: A condition when the heart stops beating
Asystolic Arrest: A state when the heart stops beating
Auto-amputation: With certain underlying abnormalities (i.e., dry gangrene), tissue will fall off spontaneously
Autoclave: A machine used to sterilize surgical instruments

B
Bagging: Using a rubber "bag" to squeeze air into a person's mouth, manually ventilating that person
Balloon Up: Once inserted through the urethra, the tip of a Foley has a balloon that is inflated in the bladder, to anchor the catheter
Basilar Infarct: A stroke
Bicarb: Bicarbonate, a measure of blood acid levels, normal is approx 25
Big and Yellow: A patient with fluid in the belly (ascites) and jaundice
Bigelow: A floor in MGH

Bigelow 8: Formerly, the floor at MGH on which the MICU was located

Bigelow 9: The building and floor number in the MGH that houses the MICU

Bilateral: Both sides

BKA: Below the knee amputation

Blacker than red: Indicating poor blood oxygen levels

Blakemore: Short for Sengstaken-Blakemore Tube, a device to stop bleeding from the esophagus

Blood Gas: Arterial Blood Gas, a blood test measuring how well a person is getting oxygen into the blood

Blood sugar of 29: Normal levels are 80-120. Insulin lowers the blood sugar

Blue Books: Books containing patient medication lists

Books for Rounds: Medical charts and vital sign sheets

BP of 40: Blood Pressure of 40 mm Hg, with normal being 100-140 mm Hg

Brain Dead: A medical or legal term indicating loss of cognitive brain function

Bronchitis: An infection or inflammation of the upper airways

Bronchus: An air passage in the lungs

Buff: Slang, to treat a patient, correcting any abnormalities

Bulfinch: The original MGH building

Bulfinch ICU: Preceding the current MICU, in a different building in MGH

C

CABG: Coronary artery bypass graft, or heart bypass surgery (e.g., of 3 vessels)

Cachectic: Emaciated

CAD: Coronary artery disease, or heart disease

Calcium-Channel Blockers: Blood pressure medications, also used to treat pulmonary hypertension

Call Days: At the time, residents were on call (stayed overnight in the hospital in addition to their usual daytime responsibilities) every third day, or 13 times in 37 days.

Cannulate: Insertion of a tube (like a catheter) into a cavity (like a vein)

Cardiac Arrest: A state when the heart stops pumping blood

Cardiothoracic: Heart and lung

Cardiovert: To shock the heart with electricity to regain a normal rhythm

Cards: 3 x 5 inch cards on which patient information is kept

Cath: Short for cardiac catheterization

Catheterization: Short for cardiac catheterization

Cavitations: Abnormalities on the chest X-ray indicating infection

CC: milliliters

Cellulitis: A skin infection

Central Drive: The brain's regulation of breathing activity

Central Line: An intravenous line that enters the neck or chest and rests near the heart

Central Venous Pressure: A measure of heart function or fluid volume

Change in Mental Status: Alteration in ability to think clearly and appropriately

Cheech: Slang for Chi-chi, enduring injustices as a prelude to death

Chest Pain: Rated by the patient on a 1-10 scale

CHF: Congestive heart failure, failure of the heart to pump blood well

Chi-chi: Enduring injustices as a prelude to death

Chronic: A long-term problem

Cirrhosis: Liver failure

CLL: Chronic Lymphocytic Leukemia

CNS: Central Nervous System

Coagulopathic: A disorder of the coagulation system, causing bleeding

Code: Code Blue, indicating an unresponsive patient

Code Call: Code Blue, indicating an unresponsive patient

Collection: An accumulation of material, usually blood, an infection, or another fluid

Compazine: an anti-emetic
Complete Heart Block: Abnormally slow heart rate due to electrical problems in the heart
Conducting Gel: A gel required for proper use of cardiac paddles to "shock" a patient with an abnormal heart rhythm
Congestive heart failure: A condition involving failure of the heart to pump blood effectively
COPD: Chronic Obstructive Pulmonary Disease, a lung disease which includes emphysema
Coronary Artery Disease: Heart disease
Co-sign: An MD's signature, which must accompany any order
Costochondral Junctions: Where the ribs meet the breast bone
CPR: Cardiopulmonary Resuscitation, a technique involving chest compressions
Creatinine: A measure of kidney function, normal is less than 1.4
CT Scans: Computerized Tomography X-rays
Crump: Slang, crash, go down the tubes
Culture: Obtain fluid or tissue samples to test for infection
CVA: Cerebral Vascular Accident, or stroke
CVVH: Continuous Veno-Venous Hemodialysis, a dialysis technique for patients with low blood pressure
Cystic Fibrosis: An inherited disease with mucus build-up and chronic lung infections

D
DC: Discharge or discontinue
Death Star: Slang, the MGH MICU
Decorticate: A body position indicating loss of all but the most basic of brain functions
Defibrillator: The cardiac paddles, which use electricity to treat abnormal rhythms
Delta Waves: Patterns of electrical activity on an EEG
Depruned: Slang, rehydrated

Differential Diagnosis: A list of potential causes of a disorder

Dispo: Disposition, discharge planning, or where the patient will go when leaving the ICU

DKA: Diabetic Ketoacidosis, high blood sugar in a diabetic that can cause coma

DNR: Do Not Resuscitate

Dobutamine, Captopril, IV TNG, Bumex: Heart and blood pressure medications

Dog Show: Slang for multiple procedures being performed, often futile

Drips: Intravenously administered medications

DVT: Deep Venous Thrombosis, a blood clot

E

ECMO: Extra-corporeal Membranous Oxygenation, a machine that bypasses the lungs, providing mechanical oxygenation

EEG: Electroencephalogram, a test to measure brain activity

Ejection Fraction: A measure of heart performance. Normal values are greater than 60%.

EKG: Electrocardiogram, recording the heart's electrical impulses

EKG Leads: The wires that attach to the chest, connected to an electrocardiogram machine

Electroencephalogram: A test (machine) to measure brain activity

Embolic Stroke: A stroke from a blood clot or bacteria that goes to the brain

EMT: Emergency Medical Technician, ambulance operators

Endocarditis: An infection of the heart valves

Endocrinology: The study of hormonal secretions

Endotracheal Tube: The plastic breathing tube attached to a ventilator

Epidural: Outside the dura mater, the tissue that surrounds the brain and spinal cord

Epinephrine: A high-potency heart and blood pressure medication

Ethics Rounds: Also, "Autognosis Rounds." See forward

ET Tube: Endotracheal Tube
EW: Emergency Ward
Extubate: To remove a breathing tube; to no longer require a ventilator

F
Femoral Artery: A large blood vessel near the groin
Fibrotic Lung: An end-stage lung disease
Films: X-ray films
FIO$_2$: Fractional Inspired Oxygen, the percent oxygen a ventilator delivers. In air, 21%, though the machine can deliver up to 100%
Fleets Enema: A mild enema
Flog: Slang, to perform many procedures on a person without hope of ultimately changing outcome
Flow Sheets: Contain vital signs, measurements of heart function, machine settings
Fly: Slang, indicating a patient in healthy enough to leave the MICU
Foley: A urine catheter
Formaldehyde Drip: Intravenous formaldehyde, the chemical used to preserve organs after death
Full Court Press: An analogy to a basketball strategy, doing everything technologically possible to treat an illness and extend life.

G
Gas: Short for arterial blood gas, a blood test measuring how well a person is getting oxygen into the blood.
Gastroparesis: A state of inadequate stomach emptying
Gel: A gel required for proper use of cardiac paddles to "shock" a patient's heart into a normal rhythm
Genome: The set of chromosomes, or DNA
GI: Gastrointestinal, the digestive tract
Gold Standard: The best test, against which other tests are compared
Gome: Slang, acronym for Get Out of My Emergency Room, meaning a sick person who will take a lot of time to treat

Gomer: Slang, acronym for Get Out of My Emergency Room, meaning a sick person who will take a lot of time to treat
Gonads: Testes or ovaries
Graft: The vessel (either artery or vein) used to replace the diseased native coronary artery
Gram Stain: A dye added to bodily fluids (sputum, blood, urine) to identify bacteria
Granulations: Healing tissue
Groin: Cardiologists perform procedures on patients' blood vessels near the groin

H
Heart Failure: Failure of the heart to pump blood well
Heart rate: In beats per minute, normally 60-100
Hematemesis: Vomiting blood
Hemodynamically Stable: A normal blood pressure
Hemoptysis: Coughing up blood
Hepatic Coma: A coma from liver failure
Hepatic Encephalopathy: Disease of the brain resulting from liver failure
HMS: Harvard Medical School student
H.O.: House officer, a resident
Hypercarbic: High blood carbon dioxide, indicating poor lung function
Hypertension: High blood pressure
Hypotensive: Having low blood pressure
Hypothermic: Having low body temperature
Hypoxic: Having low blood oxygen

I
IABP: Intra-aortic Balloon Pump, a device inserted through the groin and up towards the heart to improve heart function

Iatrogenesis: The process by which a disease or complications are caused inadvertently by a physician or by treatment

IBD: Inflammatory Bowel Disease

ICU hit: Slang, ICU admission

Iliac Crest: A part of the pelvis

I-meds: The machines which deliver intravenous medications and "beep" when the medication has been delivered completely

IMI: Inferior Myocardial Infarction, a type of heart attack

Inferior Myocardial Infarction: A type of heart attack

Infiltrate: Chest X-ray changes indicating a lung infection

In-house: In the hospital

Intubate: To place a breathing tube, requiring a ventilator

Intubated: The state of having a breathing tube, or requiring a ventilator

I/O's: Ins and Outs, how much fluids a patient receives and how much he or she puts out

IPF: Interstitial Pulmonary Fibrosis, an end-stage lung disease

Isordil: A cardiac medication

ITP: Idiopathic thrombocytopenic purpura, a blood disorder with low platelets, resulting in bleeding tendencies

I.V.: Intravenous line

IVDA: Intravenous Drug Abuser

J

JAR: Junior Assistant Resident: the second year of residency, following completion of medical school

K

Killer *Klebsiella*: A form of the bacteria *Klebsiella* that is resistant to most antibiotics

Klonopin: Anti-anxiety medication (clonazepam)

L
Lasix: A diuretic, water pill
Lead Apron: Worn by doctors performing cardiac catheterizations, to protect them from the x-rays used to see the heart
Levo, Dopa, Isuprel, Neo: Medications used to raise blood pressure
Lined: To have intravenous lines and catheters placed
Lining: To have intravenous lines and catheters placed
Locked-in State: A person who is fully aware of his/her surroundings, but is paralyzed and at most can only communicate by blinking
Lost to Follow-up: It is unknown what happened to the patient after his/her initial presentation.
Loxapine: An antipsychotic
Lung Edema: Fluid on the lungs
Lunger: Slang, a patient with a lung disease
Lymphoma: A cancer of the lymph nodes, or glands

M
MAP: Mean Arterial Pressure, a measure of blood pressure
Masked Ventilation: A specialized breathing machine that delivers oxygen to a mask, rather than through a breathing tube.
Match: The process by which a medical student is assigned a residency program
Melena: Black, tarry stool indicating bleeding in the gastrointestinal tract
Meningitis: An infection of the tissues surrounding the spinal column and brain
Mental Status: Ability to think clearly and appropriately
Mental Status Exam: Assessment of the ability to think clearly and appropriately
Meripenim, Liposomal Ampho, Vancomycin, Chloramphenicol: Antibiotics
Meta-stable: Slang, quasi-stable, sick but stable for the moment
Methanol: A poisonous alcohol

MI: Myocardial Infarction; a heart attack

Mittelschmertz: Intermenstrual pain

Mixes: Doctors (instead of pharmacists) used to be responsible for mixing, or preparing, certain medications, including high-dose cardiac medicines and chemotherapy

Mottled: Patchy, blue skin coloring, indicating poor blood supply

MSO$_4$ Drip: Intravenous morphine, used to make a dying patient comfortable

Multi-system Organ Failure: When many organs shut down or function poorly

Multiple Sclerosis: A disease of the nervous system causing a variety of problems including weakness and bladder dysfunction

Myoclonus: Regular muscle twitch

N

Necrosis: Tissue death

Neo: Short for neosynephrine, a high-dose blood pressure medication

Neuro: Short for Neurology, the specialty for diseases of the nervous system

Neurologists: Specialists in diseases of the nervous system

Neurology: The specialty that deals with diseases of the nervous system

Neurosurgeon: Brain and spine surgeon

Neurovegetative State: Coma without cognitive brain function

No Hitter: Slang, a night without any admissions

Normal Sinus Rhythm: The heart's normal pattern of beating

Numbers: Vital signs and results of laboratory tests

O

Occluded: Blocked, clogged

O$_2$ Sats: Oxygen saturation level, a measure of lung function and oxygen delivery to tissues

Optimum Care Committee: In MGH, the group of doctors, nurses, and social workers who assist with ethical dilemmas
Orchiectomy: Removal of the testes
Osler: William Osler, considered a "father" of modern medicine

P
Pacer: Pacemaker
Paddles: Short for cardiac paddles, which use electricity to treat abnormal rhythms
PA-line: Pulmonary Artery line, a catheter placed through a large vein into the heart to assess heart function
Palpated: Felt
Pancreatitis: Inflammation of the pancreas
Panhypoglobulinemia: Low levels of proteins in the blood stream
Parkinson's: A neurological disease
Paste: Short for nitropaste, for treatment of angina
PCO_2: The amount of carbon dioxide in the blood stream, typically about 40
P.E.: Pulmonary Embolus, a blood clot to the lungs.
PEEP: Positive End-expiratory pressure, a ventilator setting
Pentobarb Coma: A state of coma and paralysis caused by the drug pentobarbital
Pericarditis: Inflammation of the sac around the heart incompatible with life
Peritonitis: A severe infection of fluid in the abdominal cavity
Petrie Dish: A lab container used to grow bacteria
PGY-1: Post-graduate Year 1, an intern
pH: The blood acid level, on a logarithmic scale. Normal is 7.40, less than 7.0 is almost incompatible with life
Phillips House: A building in MGH for medical patients
Pickwickian: Like the title character in Dickens' The Pickwick Papers, someone who is obese

Pit: Slang, the Emergency Room
Players: Slang, patients
Pneumococcal Pneumonia: Lung infection caused by the bacteria pneumococcus
P.O.: Per Os, by mouth
PO$_2$: The amount of oxygen in the blood stream, typically about 100
Poly-antimicrobial: Many antobiotics
Post: Short for post-mortem, an autopsy
Post-cath: Following a cardiac catheterization
Post-partum: After delivery
P.R.: Per Rectum, to give a medication via the rectum
Prazosin: A blood pressure medication
Pre-cath: Prior to a cardiac catheterization, the cardiologist will take a history from and examine the patient
Precordial Thump: Hitting the chest with a fist to restore normal heart function
Presented: Came to the hospital or to the doctor's office
Pressors: Intravenous medications given to elevate the blood pressure
Primary Pulmonary Hypertension: A fatal lung disease
Prognosis: The prospect of recovery; forecast
Pronestyl: A cardiac medication used to treat abnormal rhythms
Psychogenic Polydipsia: The abnormal , psychologically-motivated need to drink excessive amounts of water
PTCA: Percutaneous Transthoracic Coronary Angioplasty, or balloon angioplasty, a procedure during a cardiac catheterization to remove disease from the coronary vessels
Pulmonary Edema: Fluid on the lungs
Pulmonary Embolus: A blood clot in the lungs
Pulmonary Function Test: Assess lung function by having a subject blow into a tube
Pup Rounds: Sign-in rounds, an acronym for, "Pick up the pieces"

Q

R
Rectal bag: A device placed over the anus to collect stool
Rectal Tube: A device placed into the rectum to collect stool
Red Book: The original volume of the MICU Journal had a red cover
Renal Failure: Lack of kidney function
Respiratory Arrest: Inability to breathe enough air, requiring intubation
Respiratory Failure: The inability to breathe enough air
Restraint Order: A doctor's order to tie a patient's arms and/or legs to the bed
Resuscitate: As in CPR – cardiopulmonary resuscitation
RICU: Respiratory Intensive Care Unit, anesthesiologists who assist with placing the breathing tube
Road Warrior: Slang, patient who has traveled from another hospital
RN: Registered Nurse
Rub: The sound of the heart beating inside an inflamed sac
Rule Out: Eliminate as a possible diagnosis
Run the Bloods: Analyze blood samples in the laboratory
Running the List: Reviewing the list of patients to assess what tasks need to be completed
Running The Issues: Reviewing the plan for the day

S
SAR: Senior Assistant Resident: the third year of residency, following completion of medical school
Scleroderma Lung: An end-stage lung disease
Schizophrenia: A psychiatric disorder characterized by disorganized thinking
See his Vocal Cords: A breathing tube is placed between the vocal cords
Sepsis: An infection in the bloodstream causing low blood pressure

Septic: Infection in the bloodstream causing low blood pressure

Shock: Use the cardiac paddles to treat abnormal rhythms

Sick Sinus Syndrome: An abnormality of the sinus node in the heart, causing irregular heart rhythms

Sleep Apnea: A condition in which people stop breathing for periods of time while sleeping

Slow Code: Going through the motions of CPR and a code blue in a patient with little chance of meaningful recovery

S.O.A.P.: An acronym for the content of a daily note in a patient's chart – Subjective (what the patient reports feeling), Objective (physical exam, vital signs, labs), Assessment (What the doctor thinks is transpiring), and Plan (the plan for the day)

SOB: Acronym for Short of Breath

Soft: Slang, unlikely as a diagnosis

S/P: Status-post, the state following

Spikes: To have a fever

Splenic Abscess: An infection of the spleen

Sputum: Phlegm, mucus

Squirrelly: Difficult to qualify; atypical

Status: Meaning a "Do Not Resuscitate or Intubate" agreement

Status-post: The state following

Sternum: Breast bone

Stroked-out: Slang, a patient who has had a stroke

Subclavian Line: An intravenous line into the subclavian vein, in the chest

Sub-intern: A fourth-year medical student

Suprapubic Tube: A bladder or urinary catheter (like a Foley) that enters via a hole in the lower abdomen

SVT: An abnormal cardiac rhythm, supraventricular tachycardia

Swing: The resident responsible for ordering tests, calling consulting physicians, and performing procedures on all MICU patients on a given day

Syncope: A fainting episode

T
Tachycardia: Fast beating of the heart
Tachyphylaxis: Diminished response to a drug after repetitive administration
Tamponade: Occurs when fluid in the sac surrounding the heart restricts the heart's normal function
Tap: To insert a needle and withdraw a sample of fluid
TB: Tuberculosis
TBB: Total Body Balance, the net of the amount of fluids a person has taken in minus the amount put out
Techs: Respiratory therapists or Nurse's Aids
'tern: Intern
Texas Catheter: A urinary catheter that fits over the penis like a condom
The T: Short for MBTA, Metropolitan Boston Transit Authority subway
The Tube: The plastic breathing tube attached to a ventilator
Tissue Perfusion Pressure: A measure of the amount of blood perfusing the organs
Tmax: The highest temperature in a 24 hour period
TNG, Inderal, Heparin: Medications to treat angina
TSH: Thyroid Stimulating Hormone, which provokes the thyroid to function.
Toxic: Slang, at the breaking point, on the edge, angry
Toxicology Screen: Blood test for drug or poison levels
Trach: Short for tracheostomy, a breathing tube inserted through the front of the neck
Trached: With a tracheostomy, a breathing tube inserted through the front of the neck
Train Wreck: Slang for a very sick patient
Transvenous Pacer: An emergency pacemaker, placed outside of the body with wires threaded through veins into the heart
Trendelenberg: A bed position with the head lower than the feet, in an effort to deliver more blood to the brain

Tube: The plastic breathing tube attached to a ventilator
Tubing: Slang, to place a breathing tube; to intubate

U
Ureteral Obstruction: Blockage of the ureters, which connect the kidneys to the bladder
Urinary Retention: The keeping in the bladder of urine, which normally should be discharged
Urology: Specialists in the genitourinary organs
UTI: Urinary Tract Infection

V
VA: Veterans Administration
Valproate: Mood stabilizing or seizure medication
Varices: Dilated veins in the esophagus, or swallowing tube, from liver failure, that have a tendency to bleed
Vegetations: Bacteria on a heart valve
Vent: Ventilator machine, respirator
Vent-dependent: Relying on a ventilator
Vented: On the ventilator
Ventilating: On the ventilator
VF: An abnormal rhythm, ventricular fibrillation
VF Arrest: A state when the heart stops pumping blood because of an abnormal rhythm, ventricular fibrillation
VFibbed: An abnormal rhythm, ventricular fibrillation
Visit: At MGH, the attending physician
VT: An abnormal cardiac rhythm, ventricular tachycardia
V-tach: An abnormal cardiac rhythm, ventricular tachycardia
V-tach arrest: The heart stops pumping blood because of an abnormal rhythm, ventricular tachycardia

W
Walpole: A local prison

Walrus: A large catheter
Wean: To minimize dependence on the ventilator
Wedge: A measure of heart function
Wedge Pressure: A measure of heart function
White 8: A floor in MGH
White Cells: Short for white blood cells
White Desk: Colloquial for the Admitting Office in MGH, to whom deaths are reported

X
Xylem and Phloem: The main conduits of water and nutrition in plants
Xylo, Bretylium, Pronestyl: Cardiac medications used to suppress abnormal rhythms

Y

Z

35561217R00123

Made in the USA
Lexington, KY
15 September 2014